DOMESTIC MENTAL ABUSE

A BOOK FOR **EVERY** WOMAN

DOMESTIC MENTAL ABUSE

...BECAUSE THIS IS NOT WHAT YOU THINK IT IS!

IAN CHARLES

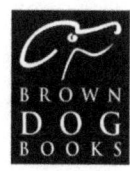

BROWN DOG BOOKS

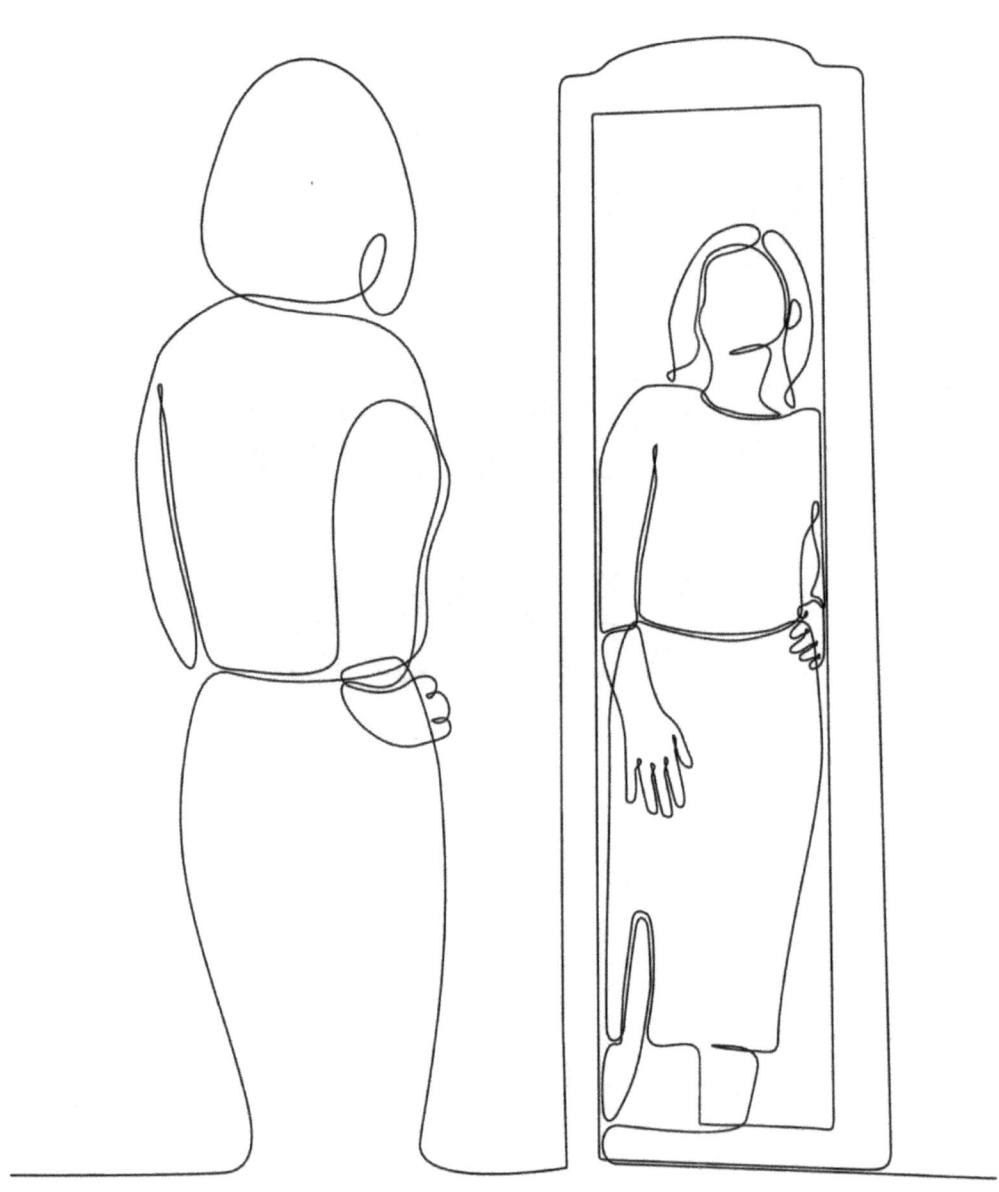

This book is dedicated to the women who shared their stories and the people who contributed their research and understanding to make it possible. They have all helped to create a unique opportunity for women to save themselves from this underhand and secretive side of human nature.

It is also dedicated to my beautiful wife, whose drive and backing pushed it to completion and publishing. We believe this new information can help any woman create a better life, not just those who need to free themselves from domestic mental abuse.

First published 2023
Copyright © Ian Charles 2023

The right of Ian Charles to be identified as the author of this work has been asserted in accordance with the Copyright, Designs & Patents Act 1988.

All rights reserved. No part of this book may be reproduced, stored in a retrieval system, or transmitted in any form or by any means, electronic, electrostatic, magnetic tape, mechanical, photocopying, recording or otherwise, without the written permission of the copyright holder.

Please read the complete disclaimer at the end of this book, any claims against the author or information in this book will be regarded on the understanding that the disclaimer has been read before reading this book.

Published under licence by Brown Dog Books and
The Self-Publishing Partnership Ltd, 10b Greenway Farm, Bath Rd, Wick,
nr. Bath BS30 5RL

www.selfpublishingpartnership.co.uk

ISBN printed book: 978-1-83952-591-9
ISBN e-book: 978-1-83952-592-6

Cover design by Kevin Rylands
Internal design by Andrew Easton
p4 illustration by Amar Zoni via Vecteezy.com
Back cover photo by Carli Dryburgh

Printed and bound in the UK

This book is printed on FSC® certified paper

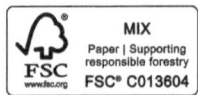

domesticmentalabuse.com

CONTENTS

Preface		9
Introduction		15
Chapter 1	A Book for Every Woman	31
Chapter 2	The Inner Abuser	59
Part 1	Who Chooses Your Thoughts?	59
Part 2	Brainwashing	90
Chapter 3	Reasons and Excuses	102
Chapter 4	Recognising the (Hidden) Signs of DMA	112
Chapter 5	Understanding an Abusive Partner	146
Chapter 6	If You Want to Overcome DMA … You Need to Change	174
Chapter 7	What Feeds the Effects of DMA and What Starves Them?	187
Chapter 8	Getting Away, Staying Away	211
Chapter 9	Leaving	222
Part 1	Leaving Mentally	222
Part 2	Leaving Physically	237
Chapter 10	Getting Ready to Start the Mental Exercises	293
Chapter 11	A Course of Simple but Powerful Exercises	307
Chapter 12	The Exercises	321
Chapter 13	Bringing it All Together	374
Chapter 14	… And Finally	384
Chapter 15	Forgiveness	385

PREFACE

Although first created to free women from the shackles of domestic mental abuse, this book grew into something much more. It became clear that the information in these pages is a blueprint that can help all women have a better life.

As a result, you have in your hands a book that *every* woman should read at least once.

The idea was to produce something easy to understand but laid bare the reason why so many women found themselves in difficult relationships without realising what they were experiencing was actually domestic mental abuse. As you make your way through these pages, you will be left in no doubt whether your partner is using subtle techniques to manipulate your mind, or not.

This couldn't be you, right? ...

Unfortunately, this kind of abuse is so clandestine that many women just don't realise there is anything wrong in their relationship until it becomes a difficult problem to overcome. Thousands of bright and intelligent women in every corner of the globe have succumbed to the tactics of narcissists throughout the years.

The starting point was to discover how a man could control a woman by subtly manipulating her mind without her realising it. The answer to this would lay the foundations to give all women a chance to overcome mental abuse permanently.

By studying every aspect, and coupling it with information from many cultures around the world, it was possible to create a clear picture of the origins of mental abuse. After that, cutting-edge scientific studies which show how our emotions can be triggered and manipulated by others had to be researched.

Then, once the root cause was exposed, it was possible to create a formula, that if used correctly could undo all the harm mental abuse can cause to a woman's mind.

The surprising thing is, this formula can be used to improve *every* woman's life by making bad decisions a thing of the past. You don't have to be affected by mental abuse to use this information. How different could things be if you never made another bad decision in your life?

You will discover what makes a woman susceptible to the manipulation of a narcissist, and how everyone is vulnerable to this until we learn how to recognise it.

This book will teach you how to do that.

Once you master the simple techniques to regain control of your life, you can choose the right direction from that moment on. No one's influence, bad advice, or manipulation will sidetrack you again.

As the book evolved it became clear it was not only women in an abusive relationship that would benefit. *Every* woman will discover something about themselves they have been unaware of until now. This 'something' not only exists in every woman but also in every man. Every one of us should learn how to become aware of it, because simply knowing of its existence, can change our lives for the better.

We are talking about a part of the mind.

Learning how to deal with this problem, how to control it and how to overcome its influence can help us all change our lives quite spectacularly. Soon you will discover how to create a better life for yourself. This does not just apply to those trying to overcome the effects of an abusive relationship, it applies to all women everywhere. If you would like to have a better life, read on. Regardless of age, gender, wealth or colour, understanding how this part of our minds can influence us, and how to control it is imperative if you want to positively change your life.

Although this book was created to help mentally abused women, so many others can benefit from these revelations too. One of the key elements to understanding and overcoming mental abuse is knowing how to control outside influences on our thought processing. Remember, mental abuse is an abuse of the **mind.** We need to understand how it affects us and accept it has the ability to remain undetected while causing so much damage to our subconscious.

Discovering this *first* will create the foundation for success. If you bypass the early part of this book trying to fast-track a victory over mental abuse, you may find yourself running in circles, just as many women caught up in this situation do.

Many of us know the old saying, you are your own worst enemy, but until we discover what lies behind that saying, we could all be acting as our own worst enemy without knowing it. Trying to deal with an abusive partner, when we don't understand what's *really* going on, can be a desperate and demoralising position to be in.

However, this book is not just about the mind, it covers all the practical steps needed to free yourself from the influence of a narcissistic partner too. Laying bare the tell-tale signs of domestic mental abuse and the things that are perpetrated in plain sight but go unnoticed by the untrained eye. It will help anyone recognise the truth below the surface of their own relationship and come to terms with what they find. Then it lays out a blueprint to strengthen the mind to be able to construct an organised plan, change their circumstances and create a better life for themselves. We cannot do anything about the past, but we can learn lessons from it to make better decisions now and in the future. Life is not a dress rehearsal, it is precious, and we only have a short time to enjoy it.

To deal with mental abuse effectively, creating a clear mind is imperative. Continuous criticism confuses the mind and doesn't allow us to see things objectively. We may think it is still possible to make good decisions after being subjected to this kind of behaviour, but this idea can be a trick of the subconscious, and a result of the spell mental abuse can cast on us all. Without knowing it, our minds can be manipulated by words we are subjected to on a daily basis. Even though we believe we still have free will in these circumstances, it's seldom the case. As you read on you'll be able to analyse your own relationship, this could be a pleasant surprise or a wake-up call. Either way, it is better to know, than to live out a lie.

Some women may have already managed to free themselves from an abusive partner, but may still be tormented by repetitive memories of the situation. Many find the effort to escape these situations too exhausting and their partner's manipulation too overpowering to go on to have a future relationship unaffected by his memory.

We can give ourselves a much better chance of success by understanding what is going on in our own minds first then learning to control our thoughts to ensure a permanent victory in our own personal battle with mental abuse.

The truth is, domestic mental abuse is probably not what you think it is.

The book also covers many pitfalls a woman can face *after* realising her partner has turned out to be such an unpleasant and toxic individual.

It is never too late to start the recovery. No matter how unlikely creating a new and better life might seem, it is possible. The most important thing to change is how your mind sees the situation right now. If you can change that, you will change everything else with the help of this book.

Domestic Mental Abuse

It is important to read everything in the right order. If you jump ahead to the chapters you think can help you the most, there is a danger the whole process will collapse. It is best to discover where your mind is working against you and learn how to deal with that first. If you don't do this, the way you think presently could influence how you judge the book and wrongly suggest this won't work for you. It would be a bad mistake, the strategy in this book can work for every woman if followed correctly and in the right order.

Whether you feel you are affected by domestic mental abuse or not, putting this book back on the shelf might deny you the chance of a better life, and the reason for this will become clear very shortly.

Regardless of your age or history, by using the techniques found here you could transform your life. You don't have to be in an abusive relationship to experience the benefits. By dedicating a little time each day to the exercises later in the book, you can disperse any negative ideas that may have been introduced to your mind and overcome them for good. Go from believing you can't do anything about your current situation, to knowing you can. There is a way out.

You will soon discover what you are really dealing with in a mentally abusive relationship:

- How a partner can manipulate *your* mind and those around you too.
- What you can expect him to do in the future.
- The unsavoury things he is capable of, regardless of how you see him at present.
- What is really going on in his mind that you are not aware of.
- What you need to do to free *your* mind from his long-term influences.
- Changes you can make to help you deal with the situation safely.

- How to avoid his influence on your life in the future.
- How to make it difficult for him to influence you from now on.
- The safety issues you may have to deal with and how best to protect yourself in the future.
- How you can improve your own mind with simple easy to follow exercises.

One of the tools a mental abuser uses to manipulate your mind is guilt. This emotion affects far more women than men, and abusers use it to their advantage with great success. You will learn how to remove old unwanted guilt that may influence your conscious and subconscious mind. Removing this debilitating emotion clears your head and helps you to realise when you put your partner's wishes ahead of yours, you respect him more than **yourself**.

Above all else, relieving yourself from guilt sets you free to make decisions that empower and protect you. When a man chooses to continually abuse a woman, mentally or physically, he has also decided to break any previous agreements in marriage, verbal contracts, or any other bond made between them in the past.

This is a unique opportunity for all women to enhance their lives, and if needed, it is a guide to freedom, no matter how much you feel trapped in a relationship at the moment.

Whatever your situation is just now, you can look forward to a better life by the time you get to the end of this book. It's best to read slowly, because there is so much new information to digest and consider. Rushing to discover everything at once would be counterproductive in the long term, so try to take your time, and let it all sink in.

INTRODUCTION

Domestic mental abuse can create the illusion in your mind that you are in control of your own life, that you are not brainwashed, and that you know what you are doing, even when the exact opposite is true … and that is why mental abuse is so successful at manipulating people without them ever realising anything has changed.

This is no criticism of all the hard work, time and effort many good people have invested to help women around the world who have been affected by mental abuse. If there is any criticism it would be toward the inadequacy of society to deal with mental abuse, and in particular, domestic mental abuse properly.

Some may say that's a tall order, and I could not disagree, however, I would argue that regardless of the magnitude of the problem, it is possible to overcome, and there can be a solution. If we first recognise the impact mental abuse has on **everyone**, not just those the abuse is aimed at, we may understand the depth of the problem better.

The difficulty here is that very few people discuss mental abuse, mainly because it is seen as a taboo subject, something many people find too awkward to talk openly about. This has created a situation where many don't know what qualifies as mental abuse. What it is, what the signs of it are, why it is used, what kind of people use it and who is more likely to be affected by it, are things we should all know the answers to, but most of us don't.

There is a hidden influence in every case of mental abuse and unless we learn how to recognise it, all of us will remain susceptible to this type of abuse … **All of us**.

Believing you are too clever to be mentally abused is no defence at all. In fact, it makes you more vulnerable.

Mental abuse is a form of long-term brainwashing, it doesn't just affect the individual but those that witness it too, even when they are unaware of any ill effects. The fact is, most of us will see some form of mental abuse almost every day and will either ignore it or fail to recognise it.

By the time you finish reading this book, you will have a new understanding of relationships, whether you are the target of abuse or not.

Before we can overcome anything in our lives, we must first accept that it exists to begin with. The very nature of this type of abuse disguises itself from all but the sharpest observer. Even when some people recognise it, few of them do anything about it.

This book has been created to help women all over the world recognise, accept and overcome domestic mental abuse. Anyone who takes the time to absorb the information in these pages will experience an invaluable, and in some cases truly life-changing opportunity.

The early research focused on finding a new way to combat the ability of abusive individuals to control their partner's minds. However, the discoveries made along the way can help all of us have a better life, not just those unlucky enough to be in an abusive relationship. For that reason, there will be a sister book available in the future, based on some of the fundamental principles discovered when researching this one. As the 21st century advances so quickly, this book is already long overdue, but maybe we were just not ready for the new information until now.

Whenever you see this symbol: ⌧ it is important to take some time out to think about what you have just read

Don't be encouraged to make any hasty decisions right now, in fact, the exact opposite is advised, slow down, think about what you have just read and absorb the message properly. That's how you will transform your life, not flicking through the pages looking for an instant cure. There isn't one. Many of us read quicker than our brains can absorb the information we are reading. Flying through this book, looking for answers, won't help. Stopping to ponder certain points, taking the time to process the information, and even re-reading it if necessary is the right way to use this book. It is not about simply reading words, it's about gaining the knowledge held within them.

For the sake of simplicity, we will concentrate on dealing with domestic mental abuse in a relationship where a man is abusing a woman, however, the content can be used just as effectively to help anyone suffering mental or emotional abuse in other situations.

Regardless of your circumstances, you have in your hands the potential to change your life for the better in quite an extraordinary way, but before you find out the truth about domestic mental abuse and how it affects us all, a little precaution is needed. From this moment on, if you are in a relationship, I would advise you to read this book in complete privacy. The reason for this will become apparent a little later. Think of it as guarding against unwarranted animosity from your partner if he sees the book and jumps to conclusions. Even the most understanding man may not be too happy if he finds you are reading a book about this subject. There is also the chance you may be living with a partner who **is** mentally abusing you, and you just don't know it yet. Before you laugh off this idea, even the most vigilant woman can be deceived by an abusive man using the right words and actions to influence his partner's thoughts, emotions and feelings. I am not saying for one minute you *are* being mentally abused, I am saying you may not realise or recognise the subtle way in which mental abuse is achieved, simply because it is so successful at remaining undetected until the situation becomes difficult to break free from.

Domestic mental abuse can manipulate a woman very effectively in the early stages of a relationship because of our inability to recognise it, even when it's in plain sight. This causes changes to take place in our minds that benefit the abuser even when we believe it is our own free will making daily decisions. These implanted ideas go unhampered and multiply as the relationship progresses. Eventually, as time goes by, this allows the abuser to take control of every aspect of his partner's life. This situation is replicated in millions of relationships worldwide, and this type of abuse, using threat, pity, guilt and fear, follows the same pattern in almost every case from Taiwan to Tibet, Alaska to Australia.

Why? Because the same pattern used to undermine a woman's psyche today, has been observed, shared and copied over many generations across the world. This super-successful blueprint was created over generations to control a partner by manipulating how she thinks and has been genetically perfected over thousands of years. Eventually, this type of control has become refined through generations and has been inherited by many individuals in the present day. Generally it does not randomly manifest in people, it is born into them. The subservient role women were encouraged to play throughout humankind's history has allowed this type of abuse to develop and improve its ability to control.

At this point, you might be saying to yourself, 'Maybe that does happen to some women, but I would know, and there is no way I am being mentally abused by my partner or anyone else!'

That could be the case, but you will find out for sure by reading this book. No matter how convinced you are about the security of your relationship it's better to know for sure than live to regret this missed opportunity at a later date. It may be very uncomfortable to look back in years to come, knowing you could have saved a lifetime of heartache by working with this book when you had the chance.

It's not easy to consider you may already be emotionally abused without knowing it, but that can be the case.

Who would enter into a relationship if they knew they were going to be abused in this manner?

No one.

Who would stay in a mentally abusive relationship, if they knew that's what it was?

Not many, maybe those that were just unaware they were being abused, or those that were convinced there was no way out.

Who would enter into this type of relationship if they could spot the traits of a narcissist?

No one.

This book will help women identify these traits before any damage can be done.

It is unlikely, the millions of women around the world who now feel trapped by a narcissistic partner wouldn't have entered into those relationships if they were able to recognise what emotional abuse looked like in the first place. It stands to reason that they didn't know what to look for or how to deal with it when they first met their partner. They ended up in those relationships because the early signs of mental abuse go undetected by most of us. It is no reflection of how intelligent or switched on someone is. Mental abuse affects the mind in a way that is hard to recognise if you don't know what you are looking for.

Watching for these subtle warning signs in a new partner's personality is probably the last thing on anyone's mind in the early days. In any case, the idea that he could eventually take control over every aspect of your life, without you realising it, would probably seem absurd. The reality is though, as the relationship develops, you could already be creeping ever closer to this outcome and still not be aware of it. By the time many women realise things aren't right they also believe it's too late to do anything about it.

It's never too late though.

The key word there is 'believe'; it's not necessarily the case that you really can't do anything about it, it's just the case that you 'believe' you can't. There is a subtle but crucially important difference and this is what makes mental abuse in relationships so powerful. The construction of that belief in your mind (as a direct result of the mental abuse you experienced but were not aware of), is the reason you find yourself thinking there is no way out.

You might still be thinking, 'That couldn't happen to me! I would know long before it got to that stage!'

That kind of belief makes it easier for a mental abuser to manipulate your mind without you questioning his actions. If you don't believe something exists, you're not going to start looking for it, are you? It would seem a pointless exercise!

All the while, mental abuse could be (I'm not saying this is the case for every single one of us) taking hold of your life without any suspicion from you that it exists in your relationship at all. As you begin to learn how to spot the early signs of abuse, it's important to understand that it creates a perfect disguise within your mind from the very start of a relationship and is a lot more difficult to spot than you can imagine right now.

For the time being at least, it's best to read the book privately and keep it in a safe place, even if you are positive there is nothing you should be concerned about personally. My advice is to keep it tucked away as you either discover the truth or satisfy yourself there is no cause for concern in your relationship.

You may be reading this book innocently because you are concerned about a friend or a member of your family and believe your partner is reasonable enough to understand that, but I would still suggest not to advertise the fact you are reading about domestic mental abuse at this stage. It is a strangely emotive subject.

No matter how clever or intuitive you are, this type of abuse can often go undetected until it is described to you in detail. Even then some people will deny the facts and continue to ignore any advice. Ironically, the influence her partner's abuse has on a woman's mind, subconsciously convinces her that there is no abuse to be concerned about! I couldn't blame you if, for now at least, you find this very difficult to believe. As you read on though, the idea may not seem quite as far-fetched as it does right now.

You may be starting to understand why this type of abuse is so difficult to discover, come to terms with and overcome.

Soon you will learn how to recognise the early warning signs of domestic mental abuse, this could save the heartache these relationships can bring. Recognising any potential problems as early as possible is invaluable.

One of the best reasons to read this book is to confirm there are *no* signs of emotional abuse in your relationship. This could help you feel more secure with your partner, free from any lingering doubt concerning underlying or undetected problems.

₪

Here is a chance to … ₪
… 'take some time out to think about what you have just read'

It's Better to be Slapped with the Truth than Kissed with a Lie

Chapter 2 holds the foundation for understanding how to use this book successfully. You will learn the reason DMA (domestic mental abuse) manages to gain control over a woman's mind. The information in Chapter 2 is important. It will enable you to understand DMA properly and overcome it effectively. Even if a woman manages to escape from her abusive partner physically, there is a grave possibility she will remain uneasy and confused, not only about that relationship but also any relationship she has from then on. Being involved with a mentally abusive individual can leave long-term subconscious scars that affect you for the rest of your life.

The information in Chapter 2 will allow you to use this book effectively. Taking time to come to terms with what you discover on those pages is the cornerstone for success in overcoming DMA completely.

Chapter 4 will help you recognise the warning signs of DMA and may highlight any in your relationship. Chapter 4 also includes many defining factors that cannot be excused as 'normal' behaviour in a partnership or marriage. By the time you reach this list of warning signs, you will find you are able to look at them more objectively and be more honest with yourself if you do recognise any traits of DMA in your partner's words or actions.

After pondering over these markers, you should be better placed to decide if you have already been exposed to DMA without realising it. This could come as a shock at first, but as you continue, you will find the safest way to deal with any points of abuse on the list that may have disturbed you. It is important to know the best way to deal with an abuser without making any knee-jerk reactions should you discover your partner's true intentions. Never confront him with any new-found knowledge. Keep reading instead.

Instantly forming flimsy plans of escape is usually a recipe for disaster. Using this book to discover a successful way to deal with narcissistic behaviour before doing anything else is the best way forward in most cases.

Further on is a chapter that explains how a mentally abusive individual sees the world, why he does what he does, and why he cannot change, regardless of how many promises he makes to do so.

If you discover you have been the subject of emotional abuse without knowing it, the second half of the book is a series of mental exercises that help to create a strong positive mind so that you make the right decisions for the future.

You will need this positive mental strength to tackle the situation properly. Long-term exposure to mental abuse weakens our ability to think straight while convincing us we have not been affected by it at all.

Once you decide on a plan for your future, the strength to stick to it and carry it out successfully is needed. This is why it is imperative to begin to rebuild your self-belief and mentality before making the next move. After years of abuse, it is difficult to break free from a DMA relationship without working on your own mindset first.

₪

This type of controlling behaviour continues to thrive around the world without any obvious effort to stamp it out, and this in itself is concerning. The failure to invest in a properly structured and effective way to suppress it is a bigger problem than we realise. Meanwhile, it continues to ruin millions of women's lives across the globe. In recent years, there has been a little more open dialogue concerning DMA and while this can be a good thing, there is still not enough in place to help women individually and collectively in an effective way.

Society does offer some limited support in the form of advice, and in some cases medication, but it isn't always made obvious to us that this help is available and the funding for it is minimal at best. DMA is all around us, but no one wants to talk about it.

It seems very few people understand what constitutes mental and emotional abuse. Much of the time those being abused in this way are too embarrassed, ashamed or fearful to come forward to discuss it. All this leaves only one avenue, we, as individuals, have to learn to recognise it properly for ourselves and do something effective to tackle it, not just paper over the cracks.

To believe someone else is going to do this for us is unrealistic when you consider the minuscule attempts that have been made around the world up till now.

We have to educate ourselves if we want to find a solution. It is not just the women being abused that are affected. In their early years especially, children are at risk of bearing lifelong mental scars associated with growing up in a house where emotional abuse is part of their daily lives. An abused woman's friends and family are also affected. They find themselves having to walk on eggshells around the problem, in case the woman pushes them away in an attempt to appease her abusive partner.

People connected to emotionally abused individuals find themselves compromised, having to adapt their approach to loved ones involved in this kind of relationship. So not only does it affect the women being abused, but it impacts their friends and family too. Many people look on as they witness awkward and offensive moments in a marriage, too scared to say the wrong thing in case it distances them any further from the woman they care for.

It is an epidemic that has not been properly addressed yet. That's why most of us don't understand what constitutes domestic mental abuse, and this puts us all at greater risk. Any of us could already be affected and don't even know it yet.

Domestic mental abuse is a covert operation, secretly carried out within a relationship, and usually going unabated until it impacts a woman's sanity. Sometimes, it is only when things go too far that a woman begins to feel there is something deeply wrong, but too often this realisation comes at a stage when she also feels powerless to do anything about it.

Many women are completely unaware that the way their husband treats them is actually mental abuse. They know he isn't very nice most of the time and bullying and verbal abuse are commonplace in the relationship, but they don't know that what their partner is doing is actually mental abuse. They just think they're in a difficult marriage. Some try to leave their partner many times, but after each attempt they find themselves returning. Typically, after long evenings of constant abuse they will walk out the door vowing never to return, but before they get very far, turn around and go back. Every time they walk out the door, **something** in their head tells them there is nowhere else to go and it's better just to return to face the music.

Something in their mind convinces them to go back.

That **something** will be explained soon, and it is one of the main reasons a mental abuser can manipulate his partner's life so much, without her realising she has already lost control of it.

Is there really nowhere else to go than to return to an abusive partner?

Sadly, in an abused woman's mind, the answer is 'Yes, I really have nowhere else to go'.

Guilt, shame or embarrassment stops them from seeking help from others, leaving only one alternative, trying to escape on their own. For a woman whose mind has been compromised by mental abuse, this option is just too difficult for her to consider. That's why she stays.

That **something** in her mind keeps saying, 'There is nowhere else to go'. Too often this is the case every time a woman leaves an abusive partner, and it's only a matter of time before she returns.

Obviously mental abuse doesn't work on the body, like physical abuse … it works on the mind, and it is **something** in her mind that convinces a woman to capitulate and return to the place she knows as home. To understand why, we must first realise that it's a part of our *own* mind, manipulated by our partner's mental abuse, that ultimately calls the shots.

I ask you again:
Would any woman enter into a relationship if she knew she was about to be mentally abused?

Albert Einstein said,

'Insanity is Doing the Same Thing, Over and Over Again, and Expecting Different Results'

This means if you have already tried to solve a problem in a certain way and it didn't work ... you need to try a new way to solve it.

Women everywhere continue to return to their abusive partners while misunderstanding the real reason they are going back. They're returning because **something** in their mind has convinced them it's the only thing that makes sense at the time. They don't realise that returning to their abuser, is a symptom of the mental abuse they are trying desperately to escape.

Domestic mental abuse almost looks like the perfect crime ...
- The perpetrator commits the abuse.
- The abused doesn't realise it is happening.
- The perpetrator gains control of the abused woman's mind and her decision-making.
- The abused woman believes she is still making her own decisions.
- No one else recognises there's a crime being committed.
- The perpetrator gains complete control and escalates his abuse to any level he desires.
- His abuse has created a dependence on him, in his partner, which ensures she will not leave him.
- No matter how bad the abuse gets, she will always return, thinking it is of her own free will.

But it isn't.

This is why a different solution was needed, a definitive one. One that exposed the reason DMA is so widespread in the world. A solution that got to the root of the problem, and diminished its ability to influence a woman's mind in the first place. A solution that explains what constitutes DMA, how it works and what you need to do to beat it.

This book can be the solution if you follow it properly.

If DMA has affected you already, the book will help to reverse that. DMA subtly diminishes your self-esteem, without you being aware of it. The mental exercises you discover later have been designed to reverse that. Where DMA has trapped you, the information in this book can set you free.

By understanding DMA properly, and working to overcome the influence it has had, you can create a better life for yourself instead of spiralling downward in an abusive relationship forever.

By using this book to change our individual lives, we can enlighten others and collectively change the way society deals with domestic mental abuse in the future.

₪

Although it's not normal practice, to use this book effectively, I encourage you to mark in the margins, beside every paragraph or sentence that particularly resonates with you. This simple act is a mental exercise in itself. It will help to strengthen your mind. The intention to highlight the things you feel are relevant to your situation means you are already becoming proactive to change it. The act of marking in the margins is a subtle notification to the subconscious of your decision to regain self-control. Do not underestimate this action, and if you don't already have a pen beside you to start doing this, get one now. (If you are reading this on an electronic device, highlight the words or sentences that resonate with you.) From now on, underline any sentence or paragraph you find particularly helpful and may want to return to quickly in the future. It might feel strange at first, writing all over a book, but this action is part of the way this book will help you overcome the effects of DMA. I strongly encourage you to personalise the book like this, and for the same reason, it is better to have your own copy and not borrow one. Try to keep it close and if you need to refer to it throughout the day you can do that quickly.

ℼ

It's difficult to believe at first, but subconscious thoughts control more than 90 per cent of our wakened lives. Many people don't know this and think they are making conscious decisions most of the time. In truth, we only make conscious decisions around 5 per cent of our wakened lives.

Once you realise this, it's easier to understand how mental abuse can influence our thoughts, without us being conscious of it happening. Continuous mental abuse subtly changes our subconscious with every harmful word or action we are exposed to.

To ensure we are not unduly influenced by the words and actions of others, we have to take more control of the decisions we make in our lives and rely less on our subconscious making them for us while we are unaware it is doing so. You'll find excellent ways to achieve that later.

By learning how to watch our thoughts more often, we become more conscious of what is happening around us. As a result of these new skills, we will make better decisions, without allowing our 'automatic pilot' to make them for us.

Mastering the ability to be more mindful of your thoughts, feelings and emotions, can help you avoid getting too deeply involved in the wrong relationship. Once you have read this book and learned how to spot the early warning signs of emotional abuse, you will find it easier to turn your back on a new partner if you need to, before you get too involved and before he has his hooks in you. Until you discover the information in these pages, walking away like this may seem a rather extreme reaction, but you will soon learn that you cannot change these individuals and their abuse only gets worse with time.

The revelations here will help those already in an abusive relationship, and everyone else to avoid these individuals in the future. We all need this information because there are more narcissists around than most of us realise. If you are unable to recognise them, you are already in danger of being taken in by them.

If you already intend to leave an abusive partner, do **not** discuss it with him. This is one of the mistakes women make when they decide it could be time to go. Advice in the upcoming chapters will help avoid the pitfalls many women fall into when they haven't prepared properly before trying to escape a narcissist.

As you read you will come across some information that is repeated, maybe even several times, reiterating the same point. This is entirely deliberate. Mental abusers rely on the repetition of negative comments to change the way we feel, prey on our emotions and control us. Anything you find repeated is designed to counteract the effect that repeated daily abuse can have on your subconscious mind. Affirming repetition is used here to reverse any negative beliefs installed by a partner's continuous abuse over a long time. Positive and uplifting advice helps to reinstate a more natural frame of mind too. When you see points being repeated, they are there as a reminder, and to reinforce your determination to overcome an implanted negative state of mind. An abuser's repetition is to break you, the repetition here is to rebuild you, fighting fire with fire.

This is a process, so if you find your mind suggesting the book is too slow, or too repetitive, think about this ...

There are five years of research behind this book. It is designed to give you the opportunity to change your life for the better, not just in the short term, but forever. The part of your mind putting obstacles in your way and giving you reasons and excuses not to use this life-changing information is the part of your mind we should deal with first. It will work against you at every opportunity, and if you are in a difficult place in your life right now … it is probably the reason why. That is why we need to address this to begin with, then you can go on to reap the benefits this book has to offer.

CHAPTER 1

A BOOK FOR EVERY WOMAN

HOW TO OVERCOME DOMESTIC MENTAL ABUSE

If you skipped past it, go back and read the introduction first, it has some important information to help you use this book to its full potential.

₪

When I started researching, one of the first meaningful statements I found went something like this:

'Domestic mental abuse is such a covert operation that by the time a woman realises there is something wrong in her life, she is more likely to believe that she is the one going crazy and the situation she feels so helpless in, has nothing to do with her partner.'

The instant I read this I knew it was true. At that time, right in front of my eyes, I was witnessing this very scenario play out in the life of someone close to me.

₪

This book explains what constitutes domestic mental abuse (probably not what you think) and what it can do to a woman's mind. It also sets out what you need to do to overcome and reverse the long-term effects DMA causes.

It does this in a new and unique way. Until now, the success rate for beating domestic mental abuse and going on to have a full and happy life is low, very low. Many women have indeed managed to escape their abusive relationship physically but the mental scars remain and tarnish their ability to create a future that isn't haunted by the experience. For me, this was unacceptable, and I wanted to find a way to help women not only survive but also thrive after such an experience.

I watched a beautiful woman's life being ruined by domestic mental abuse. At the time I tried to find answers to her situation, reading books on the subject, researching on the web and trawling through forum after forum going over hundreds of women's own personal and harrowing experiences. I could not find a definitive answer or an action plan that would help a woman recover completely from an emotionally abusive relationship and I found little to explain how to escape an abusive partner safely. Getting away from him physically is not the end of the story, if you don't work on the emotional damage DMA can cause, you are in danger of inexplicably returning to your ex and more of his abuse. A woman affected by the influences of DMA will still feel compelled to return even when she is aware of the abuse he is capable of inflicting and the dangers of being in his company. It's important to know how emotional abuse can still affect your mind and your thought processes, even if your abusive partner is no longer around.

If you want to find real peace and happiness in your life after escaping emotional abuse, you can … by using this book correctly.

In my search, I couldn't find a book that dealt with all the aspects of this kind of abuse, so finally, after expanding the investigation without success, I decided to create one myself. I believe it is unique, based on numerous sources, different perspectives and intense research to find the answers to this global problem. To determine why DMA is so difficult to overcome, I explored the latest scientific studies of the brain and how it works, then constructed a step-by-step guide to help **all** women affected by mental abuse. It helps you recognise and deal with the situation physically but also explains how to create the right mindset to defeat the long-lasting effects DMA can have.

It can help you recover from the depths of the most troublesome and abusive relationship. It is precise, clear and easy to follow.

- You will find detailed lists covering the words, phrases and actions that constitute mental abuse. Some will be obvious, but many of them will be surprising.
- There is practical advice on personal safety when you are involved with someone who uses emotional abuse and fear to control you.
- There is an outlined action plan on how to leave an abusive partner safely.
- The most important part of the book explains how to overcome the change domestic mental abuse can have on your mind, and why you may not even be aware you have been mentally manipulated.

It may seem there is no need to have to explain it, but most people don't understand what mental abuse actually is. It's called mental abuse because it affects the mind, and it can change your mind, without you knowing. Reversing those changes is crucial to beating it properly. You cannot overcome DMA by simply walking out the door, it's not that easy. Many women will throw on their coats and leave amid their partner's latest tirade of abuse, but in a very short time, their minds will convince them to return. There are many women who would tell you they have done exactly that but are still trapped in this type of relationship today. Some have left and returned over a dozen times.

Until the uninformed observer discovers the reason behind this behaviour, these repetitive actions can appear very strange indeed.

If you are being mentally abused, it may be helpful to understand you are not alone even though it can feel that way. Many women across the world are going through the same situation you might be experiencing right now. No matter where you live on this earth, mental abusers operate in the same way, and the reason for that is explained later.

They follow the same pattern, use the same rhetoric and the same manipulative techniques all around the world. For that reason, this book can be used to reverse the effects of DMA, no matter where on earth you call home.

Before we go any further, take a deep breath, focus intently, and try to understand what I am about to say next …

₪

What comes now is important if you want this book to help you properly.

If you have already been subjected to mental abuse, your thoughts, and how you see yourself and the world around you will have been compromised. You may not 'feel' any different, but the inability to notice these changes is one of the major reasons mental abusers can 'control' their partner so successfully. Your entire thought process is not affected, you are still able to go about your daily routine without noticing any obvious changes. This happens while DMA influences the part of your mind that makes the important decisions in your life, and it does so without you suspecting anything. The way DMA transforms your thought processes is the reason many women find it difficult to leave their abusive partner successfully when they don't have support, help and guidance.

Domestic mental abuse is a form of indoctrination, where the subject remains completely unaware anything is happening to them. It can be implemented over months, years or even decades, depending on the intensity of the abuse. Reading this right now, **your** mind, yes **you**, could be affected without even knowing it. You may be reading this book out of curiosity, but you could be in a DMA relationship without being aware of it … yet. Using this information to discover the truth about your relationship can be quite an eye-opener, but a very helpful one at that. Your relationship may be strong and true with nothing to worry about, but the fact is, almost anyone can be mentally abused without realising it. Discovering the early signs of DMA can be enlightening, the first steps to understanding how your mind can be manipulated.

DMA can control your thoughts so much, that it may already be trying to convince you this book doesn't apply to you and there's no need to continue reading. It can infiltrate your mind and be so subtly persuasive that you do not recognise it is already influencing your day-to-day decisions.

This influence, created by exposure to DMA, is capable of producing reasons and excuses that seem legitimate to you but have been created in your mind to divert you away from the information in this book or anything else offering an explanation to your predicament.

This idea may seem like science fiction, but it is actually science fact and part of the reason mental abuse is so successful at controlling people without them realising it. It may all seem too far-fetched to you at this point, but try to keep an open mind as you continue to read. If any thought of closing this book enters your head, remind yourself, that you may miss life-changing information. The only sure way to discover if these pages can deliver is by reading them and using the techniques to ensure you always make the best decisions for *you* from now on.

Try not to let your mind assume anything until you have reached the last page. No one else, regardless of their profession, is in a position to tell you whether the mental exercises in Part 2 will help **you** change **your** life, because they simply do not know. This is a journey only you can make before judging the results properly. This book will deliver if you follow the recommendations and exercises correctly. Only the people who have already changed their lives using these techniques are in a position to advise how well they work. Anyone who has not followed the book closely, cannot expect to reap all of its benefits. Guessing whether the advice will work for you is unrealistic too. You need to commit to it all.

₪

If you are already under the influence of DMA, that part of your mind will recognise this book as a threat and will try to reject any changes you may want to make as you continue reading. To overcome this influence, be determined or curious enough to keep reading and perhaps rediscover your true self again. If DMA has changed you, be assured, that you can become the person you once were, only a little older and much wiser.

Even if you haven't been exposed to DMA, the exercises in this book can still help you strengthen your self-belief, and create a stronger, more positive mindset. It does this by removing the negative ideas held in your subconscious and replacing them with positive ones.

₪

When random thoughts appear, we never really consider why they came along, and usually just let our minds wander, contemplating things that may never happen. We can find ourselves worrying, or playing out negatively charged scenarios in our minds for no good reason and even end up angry or downhearted. This is never pleasant or uplifting. Where do these unhelpful ideas come from?

Think about it this way, our subconscious brain controls our every breath, every second of every day, although we are not aware of it, and we can be equally unaware when disruptive thoughts come from our subconscious too.

As incredible as it may seem when reading this for the first time, we have an inborn part of our mind that works against us, not for us. It creates these random unhelpful thoughts that can cause us so much torment for no good reason.

This part of our mind is a threat to our well-being, and discovering its existence plays a big part in beating domestic mental abuse. How to recognise when it takes control and how to overcome its influence are explained later.

For now, learning of its existence and the wish to discover how to ignore its influence, should be enough to encourage you to read on. Understanding how to control your own mind properly is a big step towards beating DMA. Mental abuse has an accumulative effect, the more you are subjected to, the bigger the hold it can have on you and your ability to make the right decisions when you need to.
The right decisions are seldom the easy decisions in life.

The right decisions are the ones that work towards your long-term happiness, not the ones that make it easier for you to survive another day.

When you are under the influence of mental abuse, it is difficult to make good decisions, because your mind is usually too confused to think straight and just can't concentrate enough to make the best, long-term judgements. DMA causes a bewildered state of mind, where you find you can only think about short-term survival, not long-term happiness and that is exactly where an abusive partner wants you to be.

If you have an urge to put down this book and ignore it, you are already fighting the negative influences of your subconscious mind. It may not feel like anything has happened, but that's a small, significant shift in the right direction. If you haven't felt that urge, that's good, you already have enough positive intention in you, to carry on.

Only You Know How Your Relationship Makes You Feel

Deep down, you may have a feeling that something isn't quite right in your relationship, but not aware that it could be caused by mental abuse. You will find out later how to recognise this. It may surprise you to learn that all those sarcastic comments, put-downs and criticisms you tried to ignore by telling yourself, 'some relationships are like that', were all part of a campaign to control you. Even events that seem innocuous to you, can be part of your partner's long term plan for complete dominance. He doesn't need to lie awake at night thinking up a strategy to control your life, the blueprint for this kind of campaign is inborn, it is in his genes and comes naturally to him. It is part of his subconscious and as we discussed earlier, the subconscious controls over 90 per cent of our waking lives. He doesn't need to plan anything, in his mind, the abuse seems justified and comes instinctively. He just carries it out without contemplating whether it's right or wrong, to him, it comes instinctively. He gives it no more thought than he does drinking his coffee in the morning. Most of the time he doesn't have to consider the way he treats you, it is inherent. He was born with the ability to diminish your self-esteem, bit by bit, as the relationship progresses. This slow assault on your mind is all part of a master plan. His personality has an inborn need to dominate a partner, and it drives him on to gain complete control in a relationship. The extent of the dominance he needs, to make him feel comfortable, will determine how much freedom you eventually have. Some individuals are happy with partial control but many continue working to the point where their partner has very little freedom of choice on anything in their life.

Although much of his abusive nature is organic, there will be times when he will consciously plan to create ways of abusing you too.

You will discover why he is like this and more about his character later.

In the early stages of DMA, a woman is usually in a state of denial. As a result, she may reject a professional counsellor or psychologist's point of view if their diagnosis of her problem was domestic mental abuse. Some women may start to defend their partner, change their story or even begin to list all of their partner's good points in a bid to change the conclusion.

I sympathise with anyone told they are the subject of mental abuse without realising it themselves. When you discuss your situation with someone else and they conclude you are being emotionally abused, it's a shock to hear the truth. No matter who you are, and what your background is, it's always difficult to accept a diagnosis like that.

An inability to accept that you are being mentally abused is a type of 'cognitive dissonance' – the discomfort you feel when your behaviour does not align with your values or beliefs. You may still love the man you first met and don't want to accept you are now being mentally abused by the new version of him. That conflict in your mind causes you to doubt the facts even when they are laid bare in front of you.

Even if you realise you are being mentally abused, the chances are, you're still more likely to refuse advice and remain with your abuser than plan to leave him.

That decision usually has nothing to do with good judgement and everything to do with the effects of sustained mental abuse on a woman's mind. It destroys your ability to see the world positively, and the length of time this indoctrination takes will vary depending on the exact circumstances. Regardless of the time it takes, the abuse usually follows the same pattern as it unfolds, whether it is over one year or ten years. It begins with subtle requests and suggestions and evolves into a full-scale attempt to control your entire life.

A mentally abused woman will feel she doesn't have much time to read books, but owning your own personal copy of this book, is, I believe, the best way to overcome DMA and form a plan to rebuild your life. Reading something in print impacts our subconscious and has more of a positive influence on us overall. Mental abuse negatively impacts your thoughts, emotions and feelings, and disrupts them. This book is designed to reverse that by creating a mindset where you can control your thoughts and concentrate on your own personal well-being.

There is no instant fix to cure the effects of DMA, but understanding the need to regain control of your thoughts, has to be the priority before you can concentrate on the big decisions for the days to come.

To construct worthwhile plans for the future, you must overcome your present mindset.

Creating a strong mind is the key to overcoming DMA. You cannot do this overnight, it will take some time and perseverance, but it is possible if you use the exercises in Part 2 correctly, no matter what your circumstances are right now. However do not make the mistake of jumping to Part 2 at the moment … that won't work, in fact, it will work against you.

There is no short cut during this process and trying to obtain a result quickly, without the necessary work to strengthen your mind can be a recipe for disaster. Leaving, without creating a strong resolve first is usually unsuccessful. Women around the world who have tried to escape mentally abusive partners would testify to that. Many of them have left numerous times, only to return after each and every attempt to escape. They were not mentally strong enough to deal with that challenge and did not have the unending mental strength needed to stay away.

It is difficult to overcome domestic mental abuse without understanding how and why it affects the mind so much. Once you learn the answers to that, the process of reclaiming your life becomes a lot easier.

This book is not all about the mind, but it has to include the key aspects of it to fight DMA effectively and we will cover them shortly. Any fear created by mental abuse will diminish as you continue through each chapter. Part 2 can help everyone reverse the effects of DMA if they use it properly. Working with it requires some patience, but used correctly it can deliver long-lasting results every time.

Women who are not affected by domestic mental abuse, will discover how their lives can be transformed too. A powerful mindset that ensures you get the best out of life is invaluable and we can all create that mindset using the information and exercises throughout the book. The best thing is, it is much easier than you may imagine right now and each and every one of us is capable of this transformation.

So Why Should 'Every Woman' Read This Book?

To simplify things, when it comes to domestic mental abuse, a woman could place herself in one of these main categories:
1. You have never been mentally abused by a partner and have little or no knowledge of how to recognise domestic mental abuse properly, or how to safeguard yourself against it in the future.
2. You are being mistreated by your partner, but you don't recognise it as domestic mental abuse.
3. You are already aware your partner is abusing you, but you feel trapped in the relationship, regardless of the level of abuse.
4. You have escaped an emotionally abusive relationship (although may still suffer from the mental scars it caused).

Let's look at them in more detail.

1. You have never been mentally abused by a partner, but have little or no knowledge of how to recognise domestic mental abuse, or safeguard yourself against it in the future.
Reading this book will help to ensure you never get too deeply involved with an emotionally abusive individual. You will learn how to recognise the warning signs of an abusive nature in a new partner. For the uninitiated, these men are masters of deception and able to conceal their true personalities from almost everyone around them. At the beginning of a new relationship, they can seem intelligent, charming, funny and easy-going. Regardless of how clever or intuitive you feel you are, they can still deceive you if you don't know what to look for.

This book can help to define an existing relationship and reassure you that the odd difference of opinion, argument or disagreement has nothing to do with mental abuse. It will also help you to understand that some requests your partner makes of you, may have nothing to do with a wish to abuse or control you.

You will discover that you cannot change these individuals, and you cannot make them better. Realising this, will help you walk away in the early stages of a relationship. Recognising the tell-tale traits of a mental abuser in a new partner has the potential of saving you from a life of misery and regret.

If you see yourself in this first category, this book will help ensure you don't end up trapped in a long-term, emotionally abusive relationship, your entire life.

You will also learn the subtle signs of emotional abuse in another person's relationship. It may allow you to help them avoid a life of misery before the abuse becomes overwhelming. If you don't want to get too involved, you could just recommend they read this book for themselves.

2. You are being mistreated by your partner, but you don't recognise it as domestic mental abuse.

For a woman, the **second category** is the most difficult to believe or accept. You may be in a long-term relationship and have noticed your partner's attitude towards you decline as the months or years passed. You might think he is just being difficult at times but never contemplated he could be mentally abusing you. The idea he is wilfully involved in a campaign to undermine your self-esteem and dominate your life may just seem too difficult for you to contemplate.

This book will help you determine if you are being mentally abused but just don't know it yet. Many women believe they are in the first category here, but as they read the second, some begin to realise they have more in common with this one than they thought.

It can be hurtful when you start to realise the man you share your life with is surreptitiously abusing you and that's why your subconscious mind rejects the idea long before you get the chance to consider it consciously. Unfortunately, this allows any abuse to go unchallenged, and when that happens it slowly diminishes our mental capacity to fight back. This is why domestic mental abuse is so successful at undermining a woman's desire to challenge it. It is not your fault if you don't recognise mental abuse, the fault, if we can call it that, lies with the way the human mind works, not just in some of us, but in all of us.

To begin with, we are all susceptible to mental abuse without knowing it, and if we believe 'This could never happen to me', we are making ourselves more vulnerable. By thinking you don't need to know the truth about DMA, you make it easier for a mental abuser to deceive you, because your defences are already down. In the case of mental abuse, intuition, or the belief you are too clever to be taken in by one of these individuals, is no defence at all. That is why it's best to try to keep an open mind as you read on.

The part of our brain that ignores the possibility we could succumb to this type of deception blocks our ability to recognise when we **are being** mentally abused.

Once you realise this, it is easier to understand that you need to consciously think about your situation to discover what the dynamics of your relationship reveal. You are not to blame for anything that has happened up until now, and you are not at fault for missing any tell-tale signs of a mental abuse, if indeed there are any. A problem has to be realised before you can do anything about it.

If you discover, through reading this book, that you are being emotionally abused and do nothing, things can only get worse, never better.

Even when these individuals have completely broken their partners' will, many of them are still not satisfied. In time, they turn to physical violence to fulfil their needs. Ignoring this warning and continuing to think your mentally abusive partner will never go that far, can be a sign that the abuse has already affected your ability to make the best decisions for your future. There are countless internet forums where you will find first-hand accounts of women telling of physical violence following years of mental abuse. Many of these women's testimonies show how they regret not acting sooner. You have the opportunity to act now, if you find yourself in this category.

נ

Resisting the idea DMA could exist in your relationship may end up being a huge regret in the future. Many years from now, looking back over a life of misery, and realising you had the chance to do something about it when you had this book in your hands, may be the biggest regret of all. Mental abuse can strip you of your dignity, self-belief and happiness, while creating a life of heartache and fear. It is better to discover the truth early when it takes less effort to overcome the situation. Acting now, may be the difference between a happy life and one filled with fear, sadness and regret.

You may be thinking, 'I would know if he's trying to mess with my head, I don't need to read this'. However, to assume anything at this stage could be a big mistake, there is a chance you simply don't know it if you are living with a mentally abusive partner, especially in the early stages of a relationship.

Mental abuse creates a blindness towards your partner's behaviour, it stops you from realising the reality of the situation you are living in.

3. You are already aware your partner is a highly abusive individual, but you feel trapped in the relationship, regardless of the level of abuse.
If you find yourself in the third category, there's every possibility your mind has been compromised, by long-term exposure to continuous mental abuse. It may have created a mindset that accepts the abuse as part of your daily life. It's a difficult predicament to be in, but still not impossible to overcome, no matter how resolved you are to living the rest of your life in this manner, there is still a way out if you have the remotest wish for a better life left within you. I know a woman who finally and successfully left her abusive partner in her eighties, it's never too late.

There is always the chance of a better life to lead beyond your abusive relationship, even if you just can't contemplate it at this moment in time. Remember, no one deserves to be abused mentally or physically by another human being. Regardless of any previous marital promises, when one member of a partnership imposes mental or physical abuse on the other there is no justification for it to be tolerated. In the case of mental abuse, this is more difficult to accept, it affects your thought processes and can create 'reasons and excuses' that justify his actions towards you, but no one else. I remember being told someone stayed in a relationship because they said their partner was 'sick in the head', inferring they, the abused, were looking after their abuser! Even when the abuse turned physically violent they stuck to that excuse for tolerating it. This is how strongly mental abuse can affect a person's view of the world.

Who wants to admit that they have been tricked, or feel their mind has been compromised by their partner? It is so often the case, that a woman will not allow herself to admit these things until someone helps to look at the relationship objectively and also offers support while she comes to terms with her frightening new reality.

₪

In this category, your mind creates 'reasons and excuses' for his attitude and abuse, to help justify, to yourself at least, why you can't leave him.

As you begin to realise, you nor anyone else deserves to live in an abusive relationship and no one, not even your husband, has the right to abuse you in that manner.

When you work with the mental exercises at the end of this book, you will begin to look at life differently and your mind will start to emerge from the virtual prison (created by mental abuse) it is in. The woman in her eighties successfully left her long-term abusive husband to enjoy freedom in the golden years of her life. It is never too late to take back control of your situation, although it is better to act sooner rather than later.

By working to strengthen your mind, you'll quickly see your relationship in a different light, realising you don't deserve to be tormented any longer and from there, you can build a presence of mind to do something about it. If you don't believe at this moment you could ever leave your abusive partner, continue reading, and when you get to Part 2, immediately start incorporating the mental exercises into your daily routine. At the moment it may help to start thinking about how much easier your life would be, away from this abusive individual. With the knowledge in the pages to come, you can start to consider a plan to leave in the safest possible way. You don't need to be hesitant about contemplating this, it's only a thought at this stage. You may be some distance away from making that plan a reality, but it's still nice to be able to consider how much easier your life would be, even if you are not ready to implement your visualisation just yet. I would always advise anyone to strengthen their mind, before putting a plan to escape their situation into practice. If you have already left your partner, use the exercises to help you avoid any ideas of returning to him surfacing in the future.

He is not your responsibility. As you read, you will learn to think of yourself first from now on.

Remember, if you are being abused in this way there are millions of women who feel just like you. You are neither unique nor alone, and whatever he has convinced you to believe up until now, can be changed. As curious as it is, emotional abusers follow the same pattern the world over. By discovering this, a way to reverse the effects of this kind of abuse has been created for everyone, no matter where they live on this planet. All you have to do is follow the recommendations and exercises, and if you want to succeed, without making any short-cuts.

No matter how pessimistic you may be feeling right now, you can change. Even if you just can't see how that is possible … it is … and you **can** make it so. You may be feeling isolated and alone, but you will discover the truth is, that your vision of the world is a result of narcissistic manipulation. By realising your present ideas of life are an illusion, you can begin to see better possibilities for the future. This may take a little time, but as long as you keep working with these exercises, it could come quicker than you expect.

Remember, feelings are triggered by emotions, and emotions are created by thoughts (even subconscious ones). Having a lot of negative thoughts could be a result of long-term mental abuse.

**Change your thoughts, Change your emotions,
Change your feelings, Change your life**

An abusive partner's attitude, the words he uses and the way he says them, are all designed to manipulate the way you think and to undermine your self-esteem. If he has managed to do that, then you can manage to change it back, and this book will help guide you through that process.

₪

One Last Thing
If you find yourself in the depths of despair, believing you are in an impossible position and just can't change it … **remember this** …

… anyone can 'believe' anything they want, it doesn't make it true. Even if you 'believe' something to be true, it doesn't MAKE it true, it only means you 'believe' it is.

Right now you may 'believe' some very negative things about yourself and your life, but it doesn't make THEM true. It doesn't mean you will always 'believe' they are true either, it just means you 'believe' them just now, and you can always change your mind, can't you?

YES, you can.

The exercises are designed to change any negative beliefs into positive ones, and soon, your mind will begin to see new possibilities for the future. All you need to do is commit to using these exercises regularly.

Through his abuse, your partner's words and actions can condition you to 'feel' negative. Any negative ideas you may have right now could be a result of repetitive mental abuse.

In a very short time, you can learn to feel more positive again.

You may think, 'It's not that easy', ... but it is, use the exercises as described and soon you will begin to realise that what you may believe is impossible right now, **is** possible.

Henry Ford said:
Thinking is the hardest work there is, which is probably the reason why so few people engage in it.

You are about to learn how to think in a way that only benefits you, and soon enough, there will be a lot less negativity in your mind and your life. Whatever beliefs you have right now can fade to become a distant memory, replaced with a much more positive outlook on life.

Henry Ford also said:
If you think you can, or you think you can't, you're probably right.

It's time to dismiss thinking you can't and discover how to think you CAN.

It's okay to daydream about what you want in life, but if you want it, you have to put a little effort in to get it.

I remember one woman, who was badly affected by mental abuse saying to me, 'I just want to be happy'.

I asked her to think about what she really wanted in her life, and what would create that happiness and she said, 'All this [her abusive relationship and the problems it was causing] to be over'.

I explained to her that to cause 'All this to be over' permanently, she would have to work on her mind, reversing the thoughts, emotions and feelings that were creating how she felt at that time.

Choosing the easy path is not often choosing the right path. There are always difficulties to overcome in life, but with a strong mind, anything can be achieved. That is why the foundations of this book concentrate on developing a strong mind, which will then help reverse the debilitating mental state DMA can create. After that, we can concentrate on an action plan to achieve a better life, regardless of any obstacles that may lie in the way.

Please take some time to consider this properly before continuing.

₪

4. You have escaped an emotionally abusive relationship (although may still suffer the mental scars it caused).
You may have managed to rid yourself of an abusive partner, but are still carrying the mental scars from the ordeal. Using the exercises later will help you heal those wounds and allow you to live a life free from the shadows of that relationship.

If he is still pestering you from time to time, you will find advice on how to stop this too.

Just simply reading this book could be cathartic. Helping you to realise others have found a way back to happiness after escaping an abusive relationship may encourage you to do it too.

Learning how to expel the memories concerning your partner from your mind will help you achieve true freedom from past abuse.

It is not enough just to 'want' everything to be okay again, sadly that won't change anything.

It is not enough to just 'want' to get away from him, sadly, neither will that.

To achieve anything good in life, we need to make a plan, we need to work our way through it, and we need to stick to it.

If you are in a DMA relationship, it's not enough just to wish for better days, or to wish your present situation was over, you **have to** go through a process to get there. If you don't plan that process and work your way through that plan, then nothing in your life will change (for the better) and you may never achieve the goal of happiness and freedom.

You Have to Make a Plan
Later, you will find an outline and recommendations to include in a plan, and you can fine-tune them to suit your circumstances. Once you have done this, make sure you follow it precisely. The human mind tends to self-sabotage and there is a very real danger of this happening if you don't write a plan down and stick to it. Writing things down is much more than a reminder, it changes the priorities in your brain, making the information stick more effectively than just thinking about it without committing it to paper. To be realistic about the time you may need to recover from DMA, think of the time it has taken your partner to manipulate your thoughts and create your present mindset. If you work with this book properly you will begin to see life-changing results

in a few weeks, and in a few months, you could be living a completely different and much happier life. Right now, try to imagine how good that new life could be.

To understand why it's unrealistic to expect instant success no matter how much you 'want' it, think about this:

After the death of a loved one we all take time to recover and find a way to carry on with our life, even the people who have a very strong will still need time to adjust to this kind of loss.

At these times we cannot choose for the loved one we have lost to return, and we have to adapt to a life without them, which most of us manage to do. It takes time and depending on your inner strength and belief it can take longer for some to adapt than others.

When you eventually manage to leave your abusive partner, it can create an underlying feeling of 'loss', unfortunately in this circumstance, you **can** choose to be with them again, and inexplicably so many women do return to their abusive partner because of this 'feeling' rooted inside them. This subconscious attraction to the man that has caused so much stress and fear in your life is 'natural', but not healthy. When we finally manage to remove ourselves from a harmful relationship, there is something inside that makes us want to return to old familiar surroundings, even when they include a highly abusive partner.

You have to remember and *note down*, that this feeling may wash over you like a tide, seemingly appearing from nowhere in some cases. This is part of the reason building up mental strength is so important, you have to be able to overcome any misleading 'feelings' that suggest returning to him is the best thing you can do. Underline this with your pen, it is one of the fundamental reasons why you need to strengthen your resolve, either before, or as soon after you leave him as you can.

*Better still, get your pen and underline this (or highlight it in colour *on your device), and start getting used to marking the things in this book that particularly resonate with you.**

You may have noticed that certain points are repeated several times in this first chapter. This is not by accident, it is by design. The way mental abuse works is through repetition, for example; if you are told every night, over and over again that your cooking is rotten, there will be a part of you that starts believing it, even if you are not consciously aware of it. Repetition can reinforce both negative and positive ideas in our minds, for now, we want to instil the ideas that it is possible to turn your life around with the right train of thought.

The stronger our mind is, the better we can deal with difficult situations in life.

DMA diminishes a woman's ability to think straight and ability to make decisions, it weakens her resolve and creates a fragile mentality. It is this weakened state of mind that makes it difficult for her to stand up to her partner, or leave him altogether.

Rebuilding your strength of mind is paramount to overcoming DMA properly. DMA is an abuse of the mind and the effects this causes have to be addressed.

It's important to work with this book regularly from now on, doing so will create a 'good' habit going forward. Failure to do this because 'you begin to feel a bit better' will result in a return to the mental state your partner's emotional abuse created in the first place. *(This is worthy of underlining or highlighting.)* Sadly, I have witnessed this all too often and you should pay particular attention to this possibility. If not, it could easily happen to you.

Even if you are not convinced this book can deliver a happier future for you, the only way to be sure is to work through the exercises for **yourself**. You can presume anything or believe anything you want to in life, but that does not make it true. To **know** if this book will work for **you … you** have to follow it. There is no other way regardless of what your mind may try to predict at this moment in time.

The human brain is easily programmed and simply repeating these mental exercises regularly, can create a much stronger mindset. There is no luck involved, it works every time.

If you have been exposed to mental abuse for any length of time, you can be sure you have been programmed to some extent, there are very few exceptions to this rule. The fact that women all over the world regularly succumb to such mental manipulation, proves it is a very successful form of abuse. This course of exercises unravels the effects of DMA and goes on to create a stronger and more positive mindset.

As long as you keep using these exercises and techniques regularly, you will not return to old outdated negative thoughts and you won't succumb to emotions or feelings generated by them either.

There is no downside to using these exercises, there are no adverse side effects, and they only change your mind in a positive way.

₪

As you read on, it will become clear which of the four categories best describes your present situation.

Remember to physically mark the sentences and paragraphs that best describe your particular circumstances, feelings and emotions. This will make it easier to find the information you need to revise the most.

The key to beating **Mental** Domestic Abuse is in the name.

This kind of abuse is **Mental**.

It is an abuse of the **Mind**.

It changes the way you **Think**.

It changes your **Thoughts**.

That in turn changes your **Emotional State** and that alters **The Way You Feel.**

The way you think and feel daily is altered by mental abuse. This kind of abuse changes the way you see the world, and to all intents and purposes, you no longer have 'your own' authentic thoughts, and you no longer have 'your own' authentic emotions or feelings either. You 'feel' different, because your thoughts have been affected. Thoughts create emotions and feelings, and all three are no longer authentically coming from the real you.

To 'feel' better, the changes mental abuse has caused in your mind (even though you were unaware it was happening) have to be reversed.

₪

Domestic mental abuse does not just affect the person targeted by the abuse, it impacts those observing it too. In particular, it has a very detrimental effect on children, especially between the ages of two and twelve and the impact of watching their mother being mentally abused can affect them for the rest of their lives. It curdles their understanding of what is right or wrong in a relationship, what they see and listen to regularly becomes imprinted in their subconscious and from there may dictate how they act in relationships they have themselves, later in life.

I speak first hand having been exposed to mental abuse between my parents, I witnessed it throughout my entire childhood and right up until leaving the family home. No one explained to me that my parent's relationship wasn't natural, I had no other relationship to compare it to and therefore believed the mental abuse I witnessed every day was normal, or at least common. In fact, for me, it tarnished the idea of ever getting married. I was a clever kid and the idea of meeting someone, falling in love and marrying them, only to end up being treated like that, was just too much for my logical mind to accept. I knew I would never treat someone that way, but the fear of being trapped like that by my spouse created a mindset that never changed until I was able to deal with my subconscious … in my forties!

My subconscious decided I would never treat anyone in that manner, but also determined that I would walk away at the first sign of abuse from a future partner. Of course, I was not aware that the state of mind I had adopted was based on thoughts generated by my subconscious. I just acted out its suggestions as they came to mind and mistakenly left several partners because of superficial misunderstandings. I was overcritical, and completely misunderstood some of the situations in these relationships.

As a child, I didn't know the harsh relationship I observed between my parents was mental abuse and I certainly didn't realise how it would affect me.

The mind works in mysterious ways. Learning to understand it better, can help us all have a better, more well-balanced life.

Children may say nothing, but they are still impacted by observing this abuse daily. Even if they don't question it, they still become programmed in some way, by what they see. Although observing the situation between my parents made me positive I would never treat anyone like that, my sister ended up quite the opposite, re-enacting it, to some degree, in her marriage.

Many women deflect any idea about leaving by saying they are aware of their husband's abuse but are just staying in the relationship for 'the sake of the kids having a father around'. Superficially, this seems fair and reasonable, if you don't take into consideration how bad the abuse is, and what impact it could have on the kids as they grow up watching it. The idea in her head, to wait until the kids are grown up, comes as a result of the mental abuse the woman is exposed to. It affects her ability to stand back and contemplate what the real options are, even after she finally acknowledges her partner is mentally abusing her.

If she wasn't compromised by the effects of mental abuse, the idea that it may be better not to have their father around than let the kids grow up in an abusive environment might come to mind easier.

In many cases, children will grow up thinking mental abuse is okay because they witnessed their mother 'accepting' it.

Mental abuse is never acceptable, and it is worth contemplating the impact it will have on young minds if you continue to live with an emotionally abusive partner.

₪

Mental abuse chips away at your self-worth and self-esteem, until the abuser can influence your thoughts and your mind even when he is not around.

₪

To overcome DMA, the influence mental abuse has on you has to be reversed ...
Working with specific mental exercises will strengthen your mind,
A strong mind can reverse the influence of the abuser.

You can work to strengthen your mind ...
... either after you recognise you are being mentally abused,
... or before anyone tries to mentally abuse you.

Prevention is always better than the cure, but the cure, thankfully, still exists and still works.

Strengthening your mind before the chance of being mentally abused can stop it becoming a problem in the first place.

₪

The goal is to grow so strong on the inside that nothing on the outside can affect your mental well-being without your conscious permission or consent.

The final stage in overcoming DMA completely is to ensure you never slip back into a negative state of mind. This can be achieved by using the exercises you will learn later and making them part of your life, not just a temporary fix ... which will not last.

Whether you feel fragile or not, almost everyone's mind is affected when exposed to DMA. This exposure and its manipulative effects are more likely to influence you to make bad choices in life. Even if you don't feel any different, the decisions you make will be affected by your past and present exposure to mental abuse. This is why you must keep an open mind, before deciding if your partner is mentally abusing you or not. Until you make your way through this book, you may never know for sure.

Discovering the reality of your situation first is the only way to do something positive about it.

₪

Please remember ... ₪ ... means it is important to stop and think about what you have just read.

CHAPTER 2

THE INNER ABUSER

PART 1
WHO CHOOSES YOUR THOUGHTS?

Understanding who chooses your thoughts will change everything. However, it may be difficult, especially if you have been affected by any kind of emotional abuse, without being aware of it. Realising you are being mentally abused is not as simple as it sounds, many women don't realise their partner's nasty attitude is mental abuse, nor do they realise the effect it has already had on their ability to think freely.

Before you go any further I'd like you to stop a moment and take a few big deep breaths, it is a scientifically proven way to help clear your mind and focus on the new information in this chapter. It may not be what you expected to find in this book, but understanding and accepting what you are about to discover is the key to creating a vision of your new future and then turning that vision into reality.

Discussing the Inner Abuser has to come at this point in the book. Understanding this phenomenon contains the real answer to the problems associated with emotional abuse and is the foundation for overcoming DMA properly. There is a lot of practical information to come, but knowing and understanding the Inner Abuser, is paramount to harnessing the full potential in these pages.

Once you learn that the Inner Abuser is the root cause of all the indecision, fear and sadness in your life, you will understand how you can start to change your life for the better.

When you look at your situation, what is it that causes you the most grief?

Your partner might be frequently insulting towards you, but the way your mind reacts to it causes the thoughts that create the emotions, feelings and moods which affect you so much. It is the thoughts _you_ have in your head, concerning _his_ abuse that creates the way you feel.

If you are being mentally abused, it means your thoughts are being manipulated. If you understand this, you will also understand that you need to take back control of your own thoughts to overcome DMA.

That is easier said than done, but not impossible and you can achieve it by strengthening your mind. Being able to choose what you think about is very important for complete recovery from DMA. If you keep having thoughts of fear, guilt, doubt or any other stressful emotion, this involuntary and 'random' subconscious default will have to change to eventually become almost always positive.

If it is your thoughts that create these emotions and feelings of fear, doubt or guilt, then to beat the long-term effects of DMA, you have to take back control of your own thoughts even the ones that appear to be generated 'randomly'. You will soon discover how to change unwanted negative thoughts into positive ones. Imagine a time when every 'random' thought you have, is a positive one!

Who would knowingly _choose_ _t_o think about something that continuously upsets them?
Why would anyone _choose_ to be upset?

The answer of course is you wouldn't. Being subjected to mental abuse causes a change in the way we think, making it more likely that we have worrisome thoughts whether we want them or not. These thoughts keep us in a state of anxiety, so if we learn how to change this destructive pattern we are a step nearer to beating DMA properly.

If your partner's influence continues to disrupt the way you think, then you are still affected by DMA, even if he is no longer around in the physical sense.

₪

Mental abuse manipulates the way you see the world, drags you down, and keeps you there. You may not realise the constant unease you might feel is a direct result of your partner's mental manipulation. Early in a relationship, you may notice the odd time when he isn't very nice to you, but it's unlikely you'll realise what's really going on. Even if someone points it out, you are likely to deny the remotest possibility it is actually mental abuse.

This 'cognitive dissonance' happens when you discover something so hurtful, or so distant from your current beliefs, you try to deny its existence. To be told you are being mentally abused and don't realise it is a difficult pill to swallow for anyone. You may not want to believe it at first, or try to convince yourself it's not true. It usually is a struggle to accept your partner is abusing your mind. You might even find you want to put down this book, in case you discover the truth about your own relationship. However, that would be a huge mistake. Discovering you are being emotionally abused early in a relationship can save you from a troubled life with the wrong man. Most of these individuals are incapable of changing their own nature.

Reading this could be a critical moment in your life, but not a very comfortable one. Find out the truth in your relationship and if you need it, use this book to help you. As you continue, you will learn how to overcome DMA, instead of letting its influence overcome you.

If you become aware you are being mentally abused, you must then make a choice; to remain in that relationship and continue being abused, **or** discover how to deal with it effectively and move on to a better life. Sadly, there is no halfway house.

Why do so many women remain in abusive relationships, when it's so obvious to others that they need to move on if they ever want happiness in their life again? Well …

It's hard to imagine but DMA creates a safe place for the abuser to 'live' in your mind without being detected, enabling him to control the decisions you make and the way you see the world from 'inside'.

₪

This creates a blindness, making it difficult for you to notice anything is wrong. If it were any other type of crime … it would be the perfect one, covering its tracks, as it continues to infiltrate your sanity.

It causes you to put your partner's needs ahead of your own and defend him even when you know he is in the wrong. Remember, the first description of DMA I ever read was,

'Domestic mental abuse is such a covert operation that by the time a woman realises there is something wrong in her life, she is more likely to believe that she is the one going crazy and the situation she feels so helpless in, has nothing to do with her partner.'

This is how *'covert'* DMA can be, it creates a mindset in your head that safeguards HIM! It can even create feelings of guilt, fear and shame when you dare to consider he is at fault.

Even though you might not recognise any signs of DMA in your relationship, it does not necessarily mean there aren't any. The effects of DMA could already be blinding you, constricting your ability to recognise the abuse for what it is, and if we don't know something is broken we will never try to fix it.

Abusers are so good at this deception, even women that recognise an issue in their relationship, don't recognise the words and actions used against them are related to DMA, so they seldom challenge their partner.

An abuser also creates 'reasons and excuses' in your mind that bind you to him, in some cases, no matter how bad the abuse gets. Everything within you that protects your partner and his actions, does not come from the conscious part of your mind, it comes from your subconscious.

Learning how your subconscious mind can be manipulated by the use of key words and phrases will help you recognise the danger signs of DMA and be more alert in the future. Presently, your subconscious could be protecting him, but once your conscious mind takes over, you become aware of the abuse making it much more difficult for him to control you in the future.

₪

At the moment your subconscious has free rein, it works behind the scenes dealing with the majority of decisions you make every day of your life. Breathing, digestion, walking and talking all happen without you having to think about doing them. Most of what you believe to be 'random' thoughts are controlled by the subconscious too.

The subconscious uses a 'library' of your old thoughts and ideas to choose the 'random' things that come into your mind. That's why you'll find yourself thinking about the same things on a daily basis. Sometimes day, after day, after day. These 'random' thoughts will affect your emotions, feelings and mood.

Very few of us are aware of this, we don't realise that by practising certain techniques, we can learn to choose the subjects for our 'random' thinking.

From the moment we wake up until the moment we fall asleep, what we think and what we do are almost entirely controlled by our subconscious mind. You should stop to think about that before reading on.

₪

The subconscious runs our daily lives more than 90 per cent of the time. We are in a way, sleepwalking through life. If we are not truly conscious of what is going on around us, it makes it easy for someone else to hijack our thinking without us being aware of it. These abusers use repetitive words to influence our subconscious, and that, in turn, controls most of our thoughts. This book will help you reduce that influence and help you to think about … what you are thinking about!

Once we become aware of any subconscious mental manipulation … we can train our minds to reject it and choose our thoughts more effectively. Eventually, those unwelcome negative beliefs, which have accumulated due to the abuse, will become a thing of the past. Taking control of your subconscious, will not only help you while you are awake, but it will also help you sleep better too.

Think about this … 60–70 per cent of the thoughts we have today will be the same as thoughts we had yesterday.

While getting out of bed this morning, you didn't think, 'I will now swing my legs around and put my feet on the floor, then I will stand up and go to the bathroom, then … etc. etc.', all these things 'just happen'. You are having thoughts about doing them, but these thoughts are coming from your subconscious, you don't need to be aware of them, but they are still happening, just like breathing. When the subconscious controls this kind of action it is fine, but when it controls the 'random' thoughts we all have during the day, we need to make sure they are going to be helpful 'random' thoughts instead of worrisome ones.

Every day, we have over 60,000 thoughts, and 90 per cent of those come from our subconscious. Even though these ideas originate in our own minds, many of them may not be good for our mental health and they are the ones that are the biggest problem.

The source of these unhelpful thoughts is a part of our subconscious mind that actually works against us. It is this part of our minds that creates the bad decisions we make in our lives and it also helps DMA to control us.

When our brain creates 'random' thoughts as part of the constant chatter in our heads, our subconscious tends to return to the same things time after time, even if it's a subject we don't want to be thinking about.

The big problem is not the thoughts themselves, but **the part of our subconscious mind that chooses them.**

₪

It is beneficial to stop reading at this point, and let this sink in. **There is a part of our own mind that works against us most of the time.** It has been the main reason for making all the bad decisions in our lives, and usually responsible for our present situation, especially if that situation is not a good one.

Now that you know this, do you want to continue allowing this part of your mind to make important decisions?

I'm sure you don't. I'm sure you see the need to change the way your mind chooses your thoughts.

Once you realise your mind can, at times, be working against you, it can change everything. It is this part of the brain that helps your partner control you with his mental abuse and that needs to change.

It is very important to learn how to control your thoughts, not just your conscious thoughts, but your subconscious ones too. Practise being more aware of your decision-making from now on and don't be rushed into anything that will make your present circumstances worse, just for the sake of an easier day, today.

It's time for you to make a choice to actively work towards a stronger mindset. This choice is not one of those subconscious thoughts that run your life 90 per cent of the time, you have to consciously decide to begin working on the way your mind operates, from now on.

As you read this, your mind should be in a state of conscious thought. This means if you decide not to work with this book to create a stronger mind, by default, you are choosing to remain in your present circumstances where nothing will change and your partner can continue controlling you through his emotional abuse.

I'm sure that's not why you're reading this book. You now know you have to make your mind stronger before everything else in your life can fall into place. The way to do that is to learn and repeat the techniques you find later. They will help to increase your conscious thinking and quickly diminish the hold DMA has on you.

נ

There's an old saying, 'She is her own worst enemy'.

If 'she' is 'her own' worst enemy, then there has to be 'two' of her, that is, of course, two sides to her, two sides to her mind. The phrase refers to 'her' doing something that is bad for 'herself'.

Why would anyone choose to do something that is bad for themselves? Well …

It is the 'side' of her mind that rushes through life, making bad decisions that makes her look like 'her own worst enemy'. We all have this 'side' to our mind, and most of the time it works against us. It is also the dominant 'side' in most cases. It overrules the weaker side, which given the chance, would come to a more balanced decision before committing to anything.

₪

Why would anyone choose to cause themselves harm or emotional upset? The answer is, that many of us are not consciously aware of the moments when our thoughts and decisions are hijacked by the troublesome 'side' of our mind.

When this happens, we allow that 'side' of our subconscious to make decisions our conscious mind would be better making.

This dominant and troublesome part of the subconscious is what mental abuse attaches itself to. Because it is stronger, it has more chance of being in control, and when you add the influence of mental abuse to the equation, it becomes stronger still. So much so, that it becomes the overall decision maker in our minds, causing more bad choices, and making us look like 'our own worst enemy' to those around us.

At that point we have a very powerful influence acting on us to create more bad decisions, then feeding off the turmoil those decisions cause. This cycle in our minds feeds the source of the bad decision making it stronger which encourages us to make more bad decisions. Some might call it being self destructive.

It is in this part of our minds that DMA creates our new 'reality'. If we allow our subconscious to run our lives too much, an abusive partner can virtually control us through it. Once you know that he manages to influence your decisions through a part of your mind that usually works against you, you realise where you need to make the changes. Changes that will stop him having any more influence on your mind.

If we become more **conscious** of our decision-making, we can stop others from manipulating us through our **subconscious**.

Becoming mindful and aware of your thoughts reduces the ability of DMA to take a hold of your mind. Later on we can work to reverse the manipulative changes it has created over the years.

There is a lot of new information here to try to process all at once. It's possible that 'your own worst enemy' already has a grip on what you choose to believe or ignore. If so, it may be a challenge to consider whether you have been 'your own worst enemy' up until now. Nevertheless it's worth posing yourself the question.

This chapter is the keystone of the book. Once you accept we all have our 'own worst enemy' within, and it facilitates mental abuse, the process to reverse the power your partner has had over you can begin. If this is not clear yet, then it is important you re-read this chapter, before moving on. Speed is your enemy, slow down and you will understand more. Realising what is really happening in your life, can change everything. Knowledge is power.

₪

This idea, that a part of our mind works against us is nothing new, different cultures around the world are very aware of it and have been for centuries. The existence of this part of the mind, this 'own worst enemy', has not been widely shared with the people in our modern Western world. If it was, we would all recognise mental abuse a little easier and be able to do something about it. The old saying, 'she's her own worst enemy' illustrates a little understanding of the two sides to our mind but it does not describe it as eloquently as an old tale that comes from Native American folklore ...

An old Cherokee told his grandson,
'My son, there is a battle between two wolves inside us all.'

> *'One is Evil. It is anger, jealousy, greed,*
> *resentment, inferiority, lies and ego.'*
> *'The other is good. It is joy, peace, love, hope, humility, kindness,*
> *empathy and truth.'*
> *The boy thought about it for a while, and asked,*
> *'Grandfather, which wolf wins?'*
> *The old man quietly replied,*
> *'The one you feed.'*

If we feed this destructive part of our subconscious, we are giving in to the worst of our emotions. This story demonstrates some civilisations have been aware of this part of our minds for a long time and knew that we should be careful not to 'feed it'. In the case of DMA, we should also be careful when someone else tries to feed our own 'Black Wolf', or in other words 'abuse our mind'. Sadly the proverb does not tell us what to do if the Black Wolf becomes too strong, or how to remove its power when it does. The exercises in Part 2 provide a way to do this.

I'm sure, like most people, from the moment you wake up until you fall asleep at night again, your mind creates a constant chatter of never ending thoughts. You may have found yourself thinking about the same thing over and over again, even if it's something you don't want to!

This can be particularly annoying when it's something upsetting. Those same old fears, worries and anxieties never seem to be far enough away, do they? A lot of these fearful thoughts can be encouraged or created by an abusive partner's influence. None of us want disturbing thoughts constantly returning, but we still find it impossible to stop them from taking over our minds.

If you are not controlling the thoughts coming into your head, who or what is?

It is *your* mind after all, isn't it? So, in theory, you should be able to decide what to think about, shouldn't you?

₪

So why can't we just choose what thoughts to have and what ones never to have again?

Most of us don't stop to consider this. We continue to put up with it, without realising there is something we can do about it, permanently. Although, it does take a bit of practise. Take time to imagine a time in the future when fearful or unpleasant thoughts have no power over you, how good would that life be?

We cannot expect things to change if we don't do something to change them. How much would you like to be in total control of your thoughts? That means an end to fear, guilt, shame or any other negative train of thought that barges into your consciousness when you don't want it to.

₪

Our subconscious influences our thought processing and decision-making. We allow too many of our thoughts to be decided by our subconscious. When we leave our thoughts to chance, they can be easily influenced by abusive partners, and that is how we allow them to gain control over us. Mental and emotional abuse gets a grip on our minds by influencing our subconscious and our subconscious runs our lives over 90 per cent of the time.

That's a large part of your mind he has the potential to control.

When we become more mindful we can change this. Becoming more conscious destroys an abusive partner's hold over your mind. Diminishing our subconscious influence also weakens the influence DMA can have.

To beat DMA we have to become more conscious more of the time.

(I urge you to highlight this phrase, it is worth keeping in the forefront of your mind.)

₪

We can never eradicate the influence of our subconscious completely, but when we do allow it to have an input, we want it to be a positive one. Every day, we repeat many of the thoughts already stored in our subconscious 'library'. When we leave it to chance the subconscious will randomly select a thought from this 'library' and run it through our mind. So when you find yourself having 'random' thoughts, they are plucked from your subconscious 'library'. Very few of these thoughts are new. New thoughts usually come from conscious thinking, and we only use conscious thinking less than 10 per cent of the time.

Most of our 'random' thoughts come from this 'library' of our old previous thoughts …

Now, this is very important …

If most of our thoughts (up to 90 per cent) come from our subconscious 'library', we need to be careful about what is *in* that library! If it is full of negative ideas, put there by an abusive partner, we *need* to change this. We *have* to get rid of any negative influences from our subconscious 'library' and create a new 'library' full of positive ones.

If that 'library' is full of fear, guilt, shame, sadness, feelings of helplessness or isolation, those are the kind of thoughts we are going to be subjected to when our subconscious controls our randomly generated thinking.

Without you being aware of it, your abusive partner is filling your subconscious 'library' with negative ideas that suit his agenda to control your mind. Remember it is mental abuse we are talking about, the ability to abuse your mind. The continuous abuse he aims at you is held in your subconscious 'library'. Eventually, there comes a time when there are very few positive thoughts left in there. He has replaced them all with notions that benefit his agenda to control your mind. **His abuse is designed to break your will without you knowing it and this is how he achieves it.**

Eventually, when he has conditioned you enough, almost all of the 'random' thoughts plucked from your subconscious, will be negative ones.

Being aware of this makes it possible to work with this book and restock your 'library' with positive thoughts.

It's not as complicated as it sounds. The mental exercises are much easier than you may think, you just need to dedicate a little time each day to them. That is all.

If we can eliminate negative thoughts from the subconscious 'library', eventually, our minds may only have positive thoughts to choose from. From that moment on all our 'random' thoughts will naturally be positive ones, with little effort on our part to create them. Our 'random' daily thoughts, will come from a subconscious 'library' full of positivity.

₪

Imagine your mind as a huge library. There are only two departments, one called 'Negative Thoughts' and the other called 'Positive Thoughts'. The departments are not the same size. In recent years the department of 'Negative Thoughts' has been getting well-stocked because of your partners abuse. Meanwhile, the department of 'Positive Thoughts' has had to give up space for all these new negative ideas filling the shelves as a result of your partner's abuse. The negative department is taking over the library.

DMA has helped stock up on negative thoughts and dispose of positive thoughts without you noticing. Until reading this you were probably unaware it was happening, day by day, as life went on for you.

This means there could be a lot less positive thoughts left to choose from, and when your subconscious picks a random thought from the 'library', it is most likely to deliver a negative thought to your mind. Thus, surreptitiously changing the way you see your world. Thus, the daily, never ending stream of random thoughts is more likely to be full of negativity.

*But … if this has happened because you were unaware of the process, it can also be reversed, now that you **know** what has been going on.*

It might be hard to imagine right now, but working with this book will soon fill the 'library' with positive thoughts once again, and it will dispose of the negative ones created as a result of the abuse you have suffered.

Right now, you can make a powerful choice to start removing all the bad thoughts in your mind's 'library', and replace them with good ones.

When this is completed, any random thought plucked from your 'library' is more likely to be a positive one.

Of course, it will take some work to achieve this, but it is possible and you can do it by following the techniques to come, whatever your present situation is. If you are having any doubts about this, they may be coming from negative 'random' thoughts built up by exposure to DMA! Think about that for a moment.

Not many of us can empty our minds of thoughts. Usually, they are continuously active throughout the day. If our minds are not involved in conscious thought, our subconscious will choose something at random for us. This happens almost every minute we are awake. At times you may find yourself wondering where some thoughts came from or how you got onto the subject in your head at that moment.

If your subconscious is filled with negative thoughts and ideas, it's almost inevitable that your random thoughts will be negative too. DMA helps to create a 'library' of negative thoughts for your mind to choose from. Now that you know this you can start the process that will restock your own 'library' with positivity.

₪

- To help beat DMA learn to be more conscious of your thoughts.
- Most of our random thoughts come from the subconscious 'library'. To beat the effects of DMA the library has to be restocked with positive thoughts using the exercises later in this book.
- Restocking the library is only half the battle though, we also need to control the part of our mind that chooses our random thoughts.

₪

1. Even though you manage to fill your mental library with positive thoughts, the part of your mind that *chooses* which thoughts you have next is still in control.
2. The part of our mind that chooses our thoughts, is what controls how we think and how we feel.
3. This is the part of our mind that has the power to control the way we see the world.

The phrase, 'she is her own worst enemy' depicts two sides to our minds, and the old Cherokee tale of the black and white wolves also shows two sides to our minds. To learn how to beat DMA, everyone should understand we have these two sides that influence us.

To make it easier to understand domestic mental abuse, I call these two sides, the 'Inner Abuser' (black wolf) and the 'Authentic Self' (white wolf).

₪

Human nature depicts that the Inner Abuser is the dominant side of our mind but now that you know it exists, that dominance is already under threat. This is an encouraging start.

The Inner Abuser:

- Makes decisions that make it easier for us in the short term but can cause bigger problems in the long term.
- Convinces us we need to make decisions instantly (knee jerk in some cases), so that we don't have time to consider the situation properly.
- Convinces us to do something, then later chastises us for making that same decision.
- Encourages us to lie to the ones we love, even when it is obvious to them. (i.e. if your abusive partner stops you from going to meet friends, and you cover up the reason you can't go by making something else up. When the excuse you invent is obvious to your friends, they become more disappointed in you, and are less likely to invite you again.)
- Creates stress in our minds and then our lives, then feeds off that stress.
- Convinces us to remain in a destructive relationship when it is better to walk away.
- Is responsible for most of the bad decisions we make in life.
- Creates 'reasons and excuses' in our minds, to justify why we cannot make the best choices without repercussions

(i.e. you can't leave your abusive partner because the kids should have a father figure. Even when they are seeing the abuse daily, and it could affect them for the rest of their lives.)

So, back to the question, if it's not 'you', 'what' or 'who' is it that chooses your thoughts?

Much of the time, it is your 'Inner Abuser' and it will choose thoughts that cause more problems than solutions. It will also cause you to think negatively by default and see the wrong meaning in any given situation. It feeds on your worries.

It's responsible for all those thoughts we don't want to have, the ones that make our stomach churn and our chest tighten. The Inner Abuser is the real source of many of our problems in life. Your abusive partner uses DMA to stoke the boiler's fire, but it is your Inner Abuser that drives the train.

To reverse the effects of your partner's abuse properly, you have to deal with the Inner Abuser first. Once your **Authentic Self** is in control, you'll begin to make better decisions in your life and they will help free you from your abuser for good. As your Authentic Self grows stronger you will start to see clearly once more.

The Inner Abuser has been described in different forms, some just refer to it as a destructive part of the ego, Dr Steve Peters describes it as 'The Chimp' in his book on mind management. When discussing DMA, I call it the 'Inner Abuser' for a reason. It is the source of the problems DMA creates.

It is the reason why domestic mental abuse can control you so effectively, and why there is no need for physical violence. When your partner can control your mind, he can control your life. The Inner Abuser feeds on his abuse and uses it against you.

The Inner Abuser is 'our own worst enemy'.

The Inner Abuser takes all of your partner's abuse and uses it to create fear, guilt, worry and shame in your mind, time and time again. It can create unhelpful feelings like isolation and helplessness. It can choose 'reasons and excuses' from your inner 'library' that convince you to stay with your abusive partner, no matter how bad his abuse gets.

The Inner Abuser will also try to sabotage a woman's attempts to leave the relationship. Sometimes it will encourage you to actively participate in the drama and danger when your partner turns ugly, even though you will feel more miserable once the 'excitement' of the drama wears off. It will cause you to lie to those who would help you the most, even when the lies are obvious. This is exactly what the Inner Abuser wants, it is aware that your friends will be disappointed by the lies and may well turn their back on you. It will cause you to actively defend your partner if others air their concern about abuse in your relationship. It will do all of these things to make your situation worse, it is a master of self-sabotage, and its influence has to be addressed if you are to beat DMA effectively.

The thoughts and ideas the Inner Abuser creates shape how you feel about your life. They become your reality and are generally very destructive.

₪

For anyone reading this for the first time, the idea of having two sides to your mind may seem far-fetched. They may even refuse to believe it.

Can we really be two separate identities in one mind?

Yes, we can, and we are. All of us. Whenever we become our 'own worst enemy' and make decisions that work against us, we are under the control of our Inner Abuser.

In the past this kind of destructive thoughts have not been your fault, you were simply unaware of the Inner Abuser's existence, and you were not aware of how to change the way your mind was choosing your thoughts.

Now you know about the Inner Abuser, you have a choice to make. Will you continue to allow it to choose your thoughts or will you choose to strengthen your **Authentic Self,** and stop letting your **'own worst enemy'** continue to run your life?

Of course, if you want to beat DMA, there is no choice. You need to take control of 'who' is in charge of your thoughts, your Inner Abuser, or your Authentic Self.

The Inner Abuser is the reason mental abuse is such an effective means of control in relationships. The last thing **it** wants you to know is that it actually exists at all. Once you know about it, and begin working to reduce its influence, big changes will start to happen in your life.

You have discovered the reason behind all those recurring, annoying, negative thoughts, but much more than that, you have found the reason behind the confusion DMA has created in your mind.

Once you recognise the root cause of any problem, it is easier to solve. In the case of DMA, the real problem is the Inner Abuser.

This book will help you diminish the Inner Abuser's power, the more you work with the exercises, the stronger your Authentic Self will become. There is nothing more complicated than that.

When we create a strong mind, it becomes powerful enough to deal with all situations, not just some of them.

If you went to the gym and exercised regularly, you would become strong enough for all situations needing physical strength. It is the same with the mind. When you exercise it regularly, you become strong enough to deal with all situations needing mental strength. It is no more complicated than this. Be careful not to let your Inner Abuser convince you it is!

This is the most difficult part of the book to come to terms with. It's unlikely anyone will fully understand the existence of the Inner Abuser without re-reading this chapter at least once.

It is quite normal to question the idea of an Inner Abuser.

'A part of my mind that works against me? Really?'

Yes, really.

Imagine if you recognised all the signs of mental abuse when your partner began, very gently, to condition your mind. There is little doubt that you would have walked away before it became much more problematic. Something in your mind kept you from questioning his odd moods, bad temper or cheeky comments. Something allowed you to believe most of that is normal in relationships. Something made you stay in the relationship, even though he became more and more abusive. What was it? What created the mindset that the best idea for the rest of your life was to remain, being abused, in that kind of relationship?

The Inner Abuser?

Until you recognise the existence of an Inner Abuser in all of us, it won't do you much good to read any further at the moment. If you don't realise that your 'own worst enemy', is the real problem, you will find it difficult to get the most out of this book. Until you accept the Inner Abuser exists, it will always have the upper hand, throwing your mind into doubt, every chance it gets.

It will stay in control of your thoughts and will continue to upset you with the same old fear, anxiety, guilt, stress doubt and confusion that it has been using up until now.

More than that though, it will continue to convince you to make bad decisions in your life, while giving you 'reasons and excuses' why they are actually good decisions.

It's a part of your mind that needs to be recognised and accepted before it can be defeated. If you still can't get your head around it, and you haven't already, read this chapter again. Understanding the existence of the Inner Abuser is the golden key to your freedom and recovery from the effects of DMA and your partner's influence.

Like 'Dorothy' in *The Wizard of Oz*, 'You always had the power in you, my dear, you just have to learn to use it for yourself'.

The power to create a new life for yourself is in you, it is not magically held by your abusive partner, you just need to work with the mental exercises in Part 2 to unleash this power and overcome the influence DMA has had on your mind. The only way you will find out how effective this can be, is by doing it. Not by listening to your Inner Abuser telling you it 'won't work for you', or listening to anyone else that has not worked with this course of exercises themselves. How could they know for sure, if they haven't tried it themselves?

There are always those who believe they know better, your Inner Abuser, friends, family or even counsellors, but until you try this *yourself,* then *you,* that is *your Authentic Self* can never know.

Being in a relationship with a DMA partner is at the very least disruptive and draining, but at the most, a threat to a woman's sanity or in some cases her life.

This book helps you to retrain your mind, empty your subconscious 'library' of negative ideas, and fill it with new positive ones. When you do this, your random thoughts can only default to the positive, not the negative.

As you continue to use the exercises, your mind will get progressively stronger, and your 'library' will have fewer negative and more positive thoughts in it. Even if you can't stop having an endless stream of thoughts in your mind throughout the day, they will generally be more positive and this will make it easier to control your Inner Abuser and keep its bad influence at bay.

All you need to do is put a little time and effort aside every day to achieve this.

Soon you will be able to dismiss any negative thoughts quickly and easily and the influence they previously had on you will become a thing of the past. The results from using this book correctly can change your life, how quickly depends on how regularly you repeat the exercises, the more effort you put in, the faster the results will be.

If you don't start working to overcome your Inner Abuser, it will continue working to overcome you.

If you haven't been physically restrained by your partner, then the ultimate reason you are in your present situation is a lot to do with the decisions you have made yourself. You may blame his abuse and coercion for this, but the ultimate choice to stay with him has been yours, even though you might not be able to explain exactly why you would make such a choice.

The decision to stay has probably been made by your Inner Abuser and not your Authentic Self, and if you don't work to change your 'decision maker' (up till now, the Inner Abuser), you could continue to find yourself making decisions that will perpetuate the situation you are in now.

One woman described it to me as, 'rinse and repeat'. She eventually recognised she was making the same bad decisions over and over again.

Einstein said something like this,
'The definition of insanity is to continue to repeat the same actions, and expect a different outcome.'

If you continue to allow the Inner Abuser to make decisions for you, you will perpetuate the life you are living right now, a life your Inner Abuser has created and is thriving on. To beat DMA you have to start making better decisions, and to do that you have to change which side of your mind is making them. Your Inner Abuser works against you because the more turmoil it creates in your life, the more negativity it has created to feed on and the stronger it becomes.

Sometimes in a DMA relationship, we can become addicted to being 'our own worst enemy'. Even if those around try to help and support an addict, it is the addicts themselves that have to admit they have a problem … before they will look for a solution.

Anyone under the influence of DMA has to admit they have a problem before they can work on a solution. Escaping your partner physically may only end up being a partial success. If you don't address the influence of your Inner Abuser properly, it will re-emerge to make more bad decisions for you in the future. You could find yourself returning to your abusive partner many times if you don't recognise and accept this. Or you might choose a new abusive partner. If you think all you have to do to beat the negative effect DMA has had on you is to walk out the door and leave your abusive partner, you'll find it difficult to stay away.

If you are still doubting the existence of an Inner Abuser and solely blaming your situation on what your abusive partner is doing to you, think about this …

- If there are times when your partner is not around, why does your anxiety remain throughout the day?
- Why do those upsetting thoughts continue to disrupt your peace of mind every day?
- Where do they come from?
- Why would you choose to have disturbing thoughts about him when he is not around?
- Could it be something within your mind that is creating these thoughts?
- If it isn't something in your own mind producing disturbing thoughts, that would imply there is something outside of your body putting actual thoughts into your head, and you are unable to stop it.
- But, how can that be, your thoughts are produced in your mind alone, so surely you have a choice of which thoughts to have?

He might always be the subject of these disturbing thoughts, but he is not the creator of them, you are, or more to the point, you are not, you're Inner Abuser is. Until you do something about that Inner Abuser, it will always create these disturbing thoughts, even when he is not around.

You may say, 'Yes, but I don't *always* have disturbing thoughts when he's not around'.

We can always be distracted from even the worst situations in our lives for a little while at times, but the exception is not the rule, and your mind can return to disturbing thoughts concerning your partner many times throughout the day. These thoughts will continue to remind you that you have to walk on eggshells, be careful what you say and try to please him as much as possible just to keep the peace and avoid his wrath.

Is that the life you want to live? Decreasing the control of your Inner Abuser gives you the freedom to think what you want, when you want. By using this book properly, you will soon be able to refocus on something more uplifting, the moment you notice your mind has wandered into a negative state again.

If you do nothing about the way your mind operates at the moment, your current situation will continue, and there will never come a time when your Inner Abuser will give up its hold on you. It is more likely to take a greater hold as your partner's abuse intensifies.

Try to recognise that the biggest problem for you, is in **your** mind, and not in his. By doing this you reclaim the power to do something about it and start to make choices through your Authentic Self, instead of the Inner Abuser. If you blame your current situation solely on your abusive partner and his actions, it leaves you **NO** ability to change it. Remember you cannot change him, but you can change yourself, and that is where the power lies.

Until now, your Inner Abuser may have convinced you that the situation you find yourself in, is all your partner's fault, and if it wasn't for him being in the way, you could have a better life. It may have convinced you, that if it wasn't for his reaction to you trying to leave, you would be able to get up, walk out the door and never return.

It's difficult to leave an abusive partner successfully when your mind is confused by his continuous manipulation. Many women have discovered this after they inexplicably returned to the man they tried so hard to escape from.

If you leave your partner while the Inner Abuser is still in control, it may urge you to leave, but then, shortly after convincing you to walk out of the door, it will create 'reasons and excuses' why you have to go back. While you continue to allow it to make decisions for you, it will continue to play cat and mouse with your mind.

Leave.
Go back.
Leave.
Go back.
Leave.
Go back.

It thrives on the upset, and as your mind gets weaker, it takes a bigger hold on your decision-making, throwing your life into deeper and deeper turmoil.

If you're not alert to the way the Inner Abuser uses its influence, it may even convince you, that you are mentally strong enough to leave, then within hours, it will give you reasons and excuses why you have to return!

You could feel that you are strong enough to leave him 'this time', but that feeling may be generated by the Inner Abuser, and soon after leaving it could be convincing you to return to your abusive partner.

You may be asking, 'Well, if that's the case, when am I ever going to know if it's the Inner Abuser or my Authentic Self that feels strong enough to leave?'

Good question, you can find the answer by asking yourself:
- 'Have I been doing anything to strengthen my mind?'
- 'Have I been seeing things differently recently, because my mind is a lot clearer?'
- 'Am I just angry enough to do this just now, because his recent abuse has pushed me over the edge, at least temporarily?'

If you haven't been regularly exercising your mind to make it stronger, it is more likely the last question is the most relevant.

I hope you have realised by now, that it is very unrealistic to believe you can overcome the influence of mental abuse in an instant.

It's extremely unlikely you can change your partner's mind, he was born like that, but you do have the power to change your own mind. The power lies with you, not with him, it always did and now you know this, you have the chance to do something about your future. **You** can concentrate on changing **your** mind and changing **your** life because you are very unlikely to change his mind. Later in the book, you will discover why the idea he could change is so unrealistic.

Recognising your Inner Abuser is the secret to beating DMA.

Unless your situation has become dangerous and it is critical that you leave right now, it's best not to walk out of the door without a plan. Continue reading and practise the exercises coming up, until you are confident that you have the mindset never to return.

Try to understand that your Inner Abuser made all of your previous bad decisions when you were not aware of its existence. Your Authentic Self was not in control of your mind back then. You can absolve yourself of any blame still attached to bad decisions you made in the past. Make a decision to learn how to reduce the Inner Abuser's hold on your thoughts from now on.

This simple exercise may help, and you can start practising it from this moment on.

When you find yourself about to make a decision, no matter how big or small, ask yourself these questions;

- 'How will this impact me in twenty-four hours?'
- 'How will this impact me in a month?'
- 'How will this impact me in six months?'
- 'Will this help me or hinder me to make a happier life in the future?'

You will need to have some patience to begin with, because the Inner Abuser will still be stronger than the Authentic Self at first, so try to play out the following scenarios in your mind …

1) What would happen if I do this?
2) What would happen if I don't do this?
3) What would happen if I do 'something else' instead of this?

By slowing down and taking the time to ponder these questions you'll begin to realise that you usually have a choice, and don't have to make quick, knee-jerk decisions to please your partner if you really don't want to.

Create a phrase in your mind that you can use when he tries to pressurise you into making a quick decision. It could be something like this:

'I am going to think about this before I make a decision and I might need a couple of days'.

Try to stick to this, regardless of his coercion tactics.
The Inner Abuser likes knee-jerk reactions, it likes rushing you to make a decision, because there is more chance it could be a bad one.

Practise slowing your mind down before you commit to any decision. This is a powerful defence against the Inner Abuser's influence. If you are in doubt, try to delay any life-changing decisions for as long as possible. Even when it looks like your delay may cause animosity from others, capitulating to what **they want** and not what **you need** can be damaging in the long term. Remind yourself, that they are asking you to do what they want, not what you want. In other words, if you capitulated, you would be respecting them more than respecting yourself. If you capitulated, it would be a sign you were being manipulated, possibly to go in the opposite direction from your long-term goals and ultimately, future happiness.

Delaying any decision will give you time to come up with an alternative to a potentially destructive situation.

This takes a bit of willpower to begin with, but you will soon recognise the benefits and that will encourage you to turn this exercise into a habit.

Take a moment and decide to commit to the exercise above from now on, it's a great step to begin weakening the hold of your Inner Abuser.

₪

Becoming more aware of the consequences of white lies can help gain trust of those that might help you in the future. At times a white lie might seem easier than the truth. Using this exercise to help you realise that just one lie, especially to those trying to help you, could have a detrimental effect on your future. If you don't feel you can tell someone the truth, say you'd rather discuss the subject at another time. Becoming more aware of the repercussions of lies, even white lies, can be very beneficial in the long run.

₪

In his book *The Chimp Paradox*, Dr Steve Peters talks about the human and the chimp, and I believe, when it seems the chimp is going to get its way he asks the reader, in so many words, to have their human brain ask their chimp brain to 'wait until tomorrow', and say to the chimp brain, if 'we' don't come up with a better plan, then 'we' will go with your idea. I believe he is saying, this is a good way of appeasing the stronger chimp brain and defusing a situation where it could have made a quick, knee-jerk, bad decision.

And going on, by the time tomorrow comes the 'chimp brain' is on another mission and that big decision it wanted to make the day before, is not such a big deal to it any more.

To begin with, you need to visualise two personalities in your mind, the 'Inner Abuser' and the 'Authentic Self'.

When people started using the expression, 'she's her own worst enemy', they were recognising the existence of the Inner Abuser, they just didn't know it at the time.

THE INNER ABUSER

PART 2

It is not necessary to know a lot about psychology to overcome the effects of DMA, but understanding the existence of the 'Inner Abuser' is imperative if you want to regain control of your mind properly. Many women refer to the way DMA affected them as being akin to brainwashing, and that is a very apt way to sum it up.

BRAINWASHING

Your 'Inner Abuser' may try to convince you that you already have control of your mind, and this book doesn't apply to you. It might remind you of all the things you do daily and question how you could accomplish them if you were 'brainwashed'.

You may be in control of certain day-to-day decisions in your life, but your Inner Abuser, fuelled by your partner's DMA, could still be calling the shots behind the scenes, convincing you that there is no easy way to improve your situation, let alone escape from it. A mentally abusive partner doesn't need to control the minutia of your daily activities, only the things that keep you walking on eggshells and subservient to his needs. It's not necessarily about all-out control, just control of the situations that matter to him.

₪

Think about the people who go to a hypnotist's show, the hypnotist asks the audience to clasp their hands and asks those that find they can't undo their hands to stand up. He then picks a dozen or so from the audience and asks them to join him on stage. They can all walk down the theatre aisle and up onto the stage quite easily. They all discuss their name, their occupation, where they live and how many children they have, etc. They all 'appear' to be awake and in control of their thoughts, and their mind. Then, by the click of his fingers they all 'sleep', and when they reawaken he is in complete control of what they do while they remain on that stage. They are all 'awake' but not in control of their thoughts and actions while he has them cavorting about and indulging in some pretty outrageous and risqué nonsense.

This perfectly illustrates how you can be so 'awake', walking, talking, discussing who you are and all the aspects of your life, while there is one part of your mind, someone else is in control of, and you are completely oblivious to it. In the case of DMA, you are in control of walking, talking and all your daily routines, but you are not in control of the decisions that matter, the only thing is, you just don't know it.

Our 'Inner Abuser' is very tricky and very persistent. For instance, and this is not a frivolous joke, it may constantly give you reasons to disbelieve what you read in this book! If you do get these thoughts, remind yourself that this book is designed to secure your future happiness, and if you are determined to beat DMA regardless of any distracting thoughts your Inner Abuser creates, you just need to keep reading.

Until now, you may have believed every thought that ever entered your head had your own best interest at heart, but now, knowing about the Inner Abuser, those bad decisions you've made in the past might make more sense.

Those bad decisions, that seemed so good at the time ... was that your Inner Abuser?

Have you ever looked at things you did in the past and thought, 'How could I have been so stupid back then?'

Your Inner Abuser was likely calling the shots.

When it starts to influence your decision-making, you can address your Inner Abuser directly with this little exercise. I use a version of it myself! No matter how good you get at remaining aware of your thoughts, the Inner Abuser will be somewhere in the back of your mind, throughout your life. In the future though, you can work to make it a lot less powerful.

When I notice the Inner Abuser influencing my thinking, I say something like this to it,

'Ah, you're back, I've caught you again,
back to poison my mind with bad ideas,
but no matter how many times you come back,
every time I catch you, I'll just reject these ideas, again and again, and again.
A hundred times if I need to, but I will never stop.'

At this point, I imagine physically throwing these ideas out of my head and I finish with this thought,

'I am grateful to my Authentic Self for being vigilant'

This exercise can be used by everyone reading this book, remember, the Inner Abuser does not just influence those affected by DMA, it affects everyone's thought processes. No matter how much you feel in control of your life.

This is an exercise you can use to loosen the Inner Abuser's grip on your mind. I know it may feel strange doing this at first, but repeating something like this every time you notice the Inner Abuser's influence will help you make good decisions more often in the future. Repeat this three times. If you can, do it out loud. The mind is reprogrammed quicker if it hears the words of your voice through your ears, rather than just thinking it. If you cannot speak out loud, write it down three times. Using this technique is not nearly as effective at reprogramming your subconscious if you simply repeat it in your thoughts. However, if your circumstances at the time only allow this, it will still have a positive effect.

Repeating and affirming these beliefs is a great way to begin strengthening your mind, to some, it may feel silly or unnatural to begin with, but that is just your Inner Abuser's attempt to stop you from rejecting its ideas. Ignore its attempt and no matter how silly it feels at first, do it anyway. You may instantly feel glad you did!

This is a great exercise to help reverse the effects of DMA, persevere with it every time you recognise your Inner Abuser's influence. You'll soon feel the difference. You don't need to know **how** this works, you just need to know it **does** work. If you don't use it, you'll never know the difference it can make. Worse than that though, you'll not be actively doing something to reverse the Inner Abuser's grip on your mind and your life.

The only effort you need to make is to practise these exercises regularly, they work at a subconscious level. You may not feel much difference in the first few weeks, but your subconscious will be changing, without you being aware of it. These changes will take place, without any further effort, all you need to do is follow the exercises and repeat them regularly.

Changing your subconscious is very important, it is here where the fundamental, positive and long-lasting effects will happen. Remember, the Inner Abuser likes knee-jerk reactions, it wants instant fixes, but they never work for the long term, to make long-term changes we need to accept it will take a little more time and repetition to achieve them.

We convince ourselves that the mind is very complicated. The good news is that it is not. If you take control and steer it down a certain path, you'll soon find it will be quite happy to take off in a new direction, as long as you hold it on course … you don't need to know how this all works in your head, just do the exercises and feel the changes taking place as a result.

When did you last discuss how electricity works after flicking a switch on the wall and the bulb on the ceiling lights up the room? You don't, you take it for granted, and like me, probably have no clue what's happening to create the light. But it does work.

The only reason you might question the success of these exercises is that you have not seen them working before. This too is the influence of your Inner Abuser creating doubt over the positive outcome these exercises deliver. Doubt is a weapon used by the Inner Abuser, any time you doubt yourself, be aware of the influence the Inner Abuser and DMA is having on your mind.

₪

Repeating the exercises in this book regularly, trains your mind to default to the positive, and when you are feeling positive, you are more relaxed and when you are more relaxed you will make better decisions and when you make better decisions your life will get easier. These exercises work every time, but like anything else in life, if you don't keep repeating them, they simply won't work at all.

That's almost all you need to learn about the Inner Abuser for now.

- If you are about to make a big decision remember to ask yourself how the decision will affect you in the days and months to come. (It is important to start using that exercise from now on.)
- How will this impact me in twenty-four hour's time?

- How will this impact me in a month's time?
- How will this impact me in six month's time?
- Will this help me or hinder me to make a happier life in the future?
- What would happen if I do this?
- What would happen if I don't do this?
- When you recognise your Inner Abuser is taking control and trying to create problems repeat the affirmation above, and finish with:

  'I am grateful to my Authentic Self for being vigilant'

Think about your mind and the influence your Inner Abuser has had on it until now.

Practise these two exercises, and try to use them regularly whenever you recognise the Inner Abuser's influence on your thoughts.

Concentrating on these two issues can help to prevent making a wrong decision from now on.

Regular repetition of all the exercises is the key to your success, nothing more. Don't look for deeper meanings, just repeat, repeat and repeat as you make your way through the book learning each one in turn. Repetition is the key.

One last thing to consider.
Even after you start to use the exercises to reverse the effects of DMA, your 'Inner Abuser' will still be the dominant decision-maker in your mind for some time to come. Even as you use the exercises regularly, it will continue to be in the background, waiting to resurface and manipulate your thoughts at any opportunity it gets, and when you least suspect it.

From now on, try to be more vigilant of the direction your random thoughts take you.

I remember one woman telling me that after doing some of the exercises in this book she decided to stop seeing her counsellor, she felt there was no further reason to attend and was feeling like a fraud, taking up the counsellor's time. She told me she felt completely cured of the effects of DMA and rarely thought about 'him' any more.

A few short weeks later, she moved back in with her abusive husband and was soon suffering his abuse all over again.

So remember, you can 'feel' cured, (in fact your Inner Abuser will encourage this feeling) but it will only be temporary if you do not keep up the daily exercises in this book. When recovering from the long-lasting effects of mental abuse, especially in the early months, no matter how good you feel, no matter how transformed you feel, you **will not be** completely free of the subconscious changes DMA has caused.

The only way to continue feeling 'completely cured' is to repeat these exercises daily. If you don't take this seriously, you could easily wake up one day, back in the same bed as your long-term DMA partner. The effects of DMA are real, even if you can't see or touch them, and if you don't come to terms with the fact your thought processes have been manipulated, you are in real danger of returning to your abusive partner.

This woman's story is not an isolated one, remember, some women leave and return to their abusive partner up to fifteen times, this is not a coincidence, it is a symptom of mental abuse just like spots are a symptom of measles.

To stop this from happening to you, you must train your mind with all of the exercises in this book, to strengthen your resolve. Your mind has to be strong, to deal with previous exposure to mental abuse.

Putting time aside each day to repeat these exercises is a very small price to pay for true freedom. Remaining alert to the Inner Abuser's influences, will help you to feel less stressed and more in control of your life … particularly after the first few weeks of doing these exercises regularly. The new feeling of self-control will be a great reward for your efforts.

₪

Marisa Peer is a very successful and renowned hypnotherapist. She has written many self-help books and has worked with some of the biggest names in sport, entertainment and industry. I remember a short story of hers, and it goes something like this; she was sitting in her car one dark, cold, wet night, watching the glow of the head torches on a group of soldiers. They were training, running up and down a steep hill, each carrying a full pack on his back. A situation that would have most of us in tears in such adverse conditions, but she recalled they were all singing, repeating the line after the first man sings it, the way soldiers do. The funny thing was, she said, they seemed to be enjoying it! Once she started analysing the situation, she realised why and explained it something like this:
The brain would initially recognise, quite rightly, that the conditions were horrible. However, when they started singing, the brain would become confused, 'It's a horrible night, I am soaked, freezing and covered in mud, why am I singing? I can only sing if I am happy. It doesn't seem right, to be happy in these conditions, but if I'm singing I must be happy … Okay then, I'm not sure why, but I'm happy!'

… and, she said, they all seemed to be genuinely happy as they slid about in the mud, carrying their huge packs to the top of that hill and all the time, singing away.

You see, the brain doesn't need to know why everything is the way it is, if you exercise it in the right way, by singing in the case of the soldiers, you can get the right results without knowing, or wondering, how you got there.

Just repeating a song out loud, over and over again made these soldiers happy, and by repeating these mental exercises, you can induce happier feelings too. Consistently repeating them will create a new way of thinking, consciously and subconsciously. You don't need to keep thinking about it, you will just feel happier, more of the time.

There is no doubt, that as you rebuild your life, you are going to have difficulties along the way, but rebuilding your inner strength of mind will ensure you are strong enough to deal with them and all the other challenges recovering from DMA brings.

A FINAL THOUGHT ON HOW YOUR INNER ABUSER CAN RUIN YOUR HAPPINESS

Keep reminding yourself of this:
YOU need to make better decisions for YOU, in YOUR life
Don't let other people make the decisions for YOU, in YOUR life
If YOU don't take control of the decisions in YOUR life
Someone (or something) else will.
Your Inner Abuser will try to stop YOU from making good decisions for YOU, in YOUR life,
It's up to YOU to recognise when it does.
If you continue to allow it to interfere, then it will continue to make bad decisions for you,
In YOUR life.

If you take nothing more from this chapter, remember, that YOU have to take better control of the decisions made in your life from this day forward. Taking back control is taking back responsibility, and that means you are once again in control and responsible, for YOU. If you don't, nothing will change, you will carry on making bad decisions, or you will let someone else make similarly bad decisions for you, leading to an outcome, similar to the situation you find yourself in now.

Give this time to consider ...
Who do you WANT to be in control of YOUR life? ...
Your abusive partner?
Your children?
Members of your family?
Your doctor, counsellor or psychiatrist?
Do you want to give up control of YOUR life, to them?
Or are you going to choose YOUR Authentic Self to make YOUR decisions?

Don't forget, every single person has an Inner Abuser, you have to be careful when taking advice from others because you could be taking advice from **their** Inner Abuser. It may be in control of their thoughts, advising them badly, and that could make things worse for them AND for YOU. When discussing your options for the future with others, make sure their advice does not suit them, more than it suits you.

The best way to be sure you are getting the right advice is to help your Authentic Self overcome your Inner Abuser.

Work on replacing negative thoughts in your subconscious and practise being more aware of the decisions you make today. Think about the consequences these decisions will have tomorrow. The power was always in YOU, YOU just had to learn that for yourself.

But admittedly it may not feel that easy to take back control of your thoughts.

So why does it feel difficult to do this?

The answer is simple. You always could do it, you were just not taught *how* to do it, until now.

If you were never taught *how* to speak a language, *how* could you communicate?

We think in the languages we have learned to speak.

We couldn't talk to ourselves, in our thoughts, if we didn't use a language to do it.

Once we learn to talk a language, we learn to talk to ourselves and from that point on, as a species, we never really stopped talking to ourselves inside our heads.

The most important thing is, what we talk to ourselves about, and that is determined by who or what is in control of our mind, our Inner Abuser, or our Authentic Self.

₪

When people make bad choices in life, and everyone can see it except them, they are being led by their Inner Abuser. Watching others do this should alert us that we may be in danger of doing the same thing ourselves, and just don't realise it. Until we recognise the existence of our Inner Abuser, we are all at risk of making bad decisions and thinking they are good ones …

'Our own worst enemy' … 'The part of ourselves we can't live with anymore' … 'The rod we make for our own back' … 'The hole we dig for ourselves' … 'Cutting off our nose to spite our face' …

They all describe the influence of our Inner Abuser … but learning to recognise all of this, is the beginning of the end of its power over us.

₪

Our Inner Abuser tries to convince us that we have to continue to stay struggling and trapped in a life we don't want.

In the case of DMA, the Inner Abuser tries to convince you that you are trapped in a relationship you don't want, because of your commitments, your kids, your financial situation or the shame or guilt of divorce. But if all of these fail, then the Inner Abuser will revert to its fail-safe, and that is ... you can't leave him because you still 'love' him and it will tell you that is the main reason you should not think about walking away.

Your Inner Abuser is capable of becoming so powerful that it could convince you that you are in love when you are not, and it is not until you distance yourself far enough away from that individual, that you can look at it objectively and recognise you have been deceived by him and your own mind.

The Inner Abuser is capable of deception to that scale ... when we become our own worst enemy.

The feeling of love may have been generated by your Inner Abuser, and you might be mistaking fear, guilt and the butterflies in your stomach for love.

As you train your brain, the truth will become clear.

However, now that you are aware of the existence of your Inner Abuser and the fact it has had too much say in your life choices, it's time to become more acquainted with another part of your mind, your 'Authentic Self'.

CHAPTER 3

REASONS AND EXCUSES

After discovering the existence of the Inner Abuser, understanding how it works, (to stop us from enjoying our full potential in life) can help us change our beliefs in the future. The Inner Abuser creates obstacles in our minds, to hamper us from doing the things we want to do which give us the most pleasure …

… 'I'd love to come to the beach, but I have to mow the lawn' …

… 'I'd really like to come to the cinema with you, but I need to iron some clothes for work tomorrow' … 'I'd like to apply for that job, it sounds great, but I don't think I'm qualified for it' … 'I want to leave him, but … [*you can fill in the blank here*]'.

Once involved in a mentally abusive relationship, the Inner Abuser will have increased its hold over your thoughts, producing more 'Reasons and Excuses' to hold you back than normal. This is not ideal, because the human brain, in its normal state, can produce enough of them without any assistance.

If you are influenced by an abusive partner, the reasons and excuses your mind creates may all seem legitimate to you. Now that you realise this, try to become more aware of them for what they are, mindsets to imprison you in your present situation. A good way to shake off the shackles made by these reasons and excuses, is to practise how to ignore them. Become aware of the ideas that curtail you, look for a way around the thoughts that stand in your way, and consider ways that will serve you better in the long run. Meanwhile, try to ignore any ideas your Inner Abuser generates to get in the way.

Most of us make up a lot of reasons and excuses in our minds, we use many of them to justify why we are unable to do the things in life we really want to, but, at the time, we don't realise we are creating a prison for ourselves. This applies to us all in varying degrees, I have friends who are not in an abusive relationship but have curtailed their lives by listening to their Inner Abuser. It convinced them they couldn't follow their dreams because their own 'reasons and excuses' were standing in the way. Instead of looking for a way around the stumbling blocks, they listened to the voice in their head that justified why they couldn't fulfil those dreams. It's a common fault of the human psyche, but it becomes truly crippling for those of us under the influence of DMA.

When a woman is influenced in this way, she doesn't have to look far for reasons and excuses to explain why she cannot escape her abusive partner. When she thinks of him, and the fear in her rises, the dreams are over before they begin.

He will have created a list of reasons and excuses in her subconscious, and without her knowing it, these rules will control her life. If she gets the offer to do something she enjoys but she knows he won't like it, her usual reply is, 'I'd love to do that, but …'.

If you have an abusive partner you probably know this scenario quite well. If you are not already aware of it, start looking out for the reasons and excuses in your head that stop you, when you get the opportunity to do something you would enjoy.

'I'd love to, but I can't, because …'
The Inner Abuser constantly creates reasons and excuses to stop you from doing the things you enjoy most in life, but when you start helping your Authentic Self take charge, it will find a way around them.

Think about some instances in the past, when you didn't get to do what you wanted, and ask yourself what stood in the way? Was there a way around the situation that you ignored?

If there is something you want to do in the future, and you find yourself making 'reasons and excuses' why you can't do it, take time to think of a way to overcome what your Inner Abuser puts in the way. There is always another way to look at any situation, remember Henry Ford, *'If you think you can, or you think you can't, you're probably right'*.

It's time to start looking for the way 'you can'.

Every time you find yourself saying, 'I can't', look at the situation and find a way to justify how 'you can'.

As always, this sounds simple but takes a bit of practice before we start to find those 'I can do this' moments. There is always a way to overcome obstacles if you look hard enough, and that's when you start pushing back the influence of DMA and your Inner Abuser, allowing you to do more of what you want and ignoring the 'reasons and excuses' that try to get in the way.

Hindsight creates regret, and regret is something we can all do without in our lives. Find the way past your 'reasons and excuses' and regrettable hindsight will become a thing of the past!

Looking for a way around these mental roadblocks is necessary to continue your journey and overcome the long-term effects of DMA. This can save you time and heartache in the future. The best chess players take full advantage of the time allotted to them, before making their move. Take some time to consider how you can get past your own mental obstacles.

In the past, when you made a knee-jerk reaction, capitulated to pressure from your partner, agreed to do something 'just to keep the peace', or told little white lies to cover up his abuse, you were probably digging yourself deeper into a hole but didn't realise it at the time.

You might remember a situation like this and no doubt, come up with pretty compelling 'reasons and excuses' why you **had to** go along with them. However, when you think back, did the decision at the time end up benefiting you in the long run? Did you really **'have to'** after all? Or was there a better way you could have dealt with the situation? And if there was, can you learn from the past, and begin taking more time to find the best way to deal with similar situations in the future?

When your mind comes up with reasons and excuses why you 'have to' act a certain way, ask yourself, 'What can I do here, to get what I want, and not what other people want from me?'

Becoming more conscious of your thoughts and therefore your decisions will help you make better choices in the future.

Look out for others trying to impose their will on you, or make you feel guilty.

As you make your way through this book, you will find techniques that will help lessen the burden of guilt associated with anyone else's reaction to your choices. They have no right to try to manipulate you, but they may try anyway. You are not in the wrong … they are.

There's a phrase I came across that helps to alleviate any perceived guilt; 'What other people think of me is none of my business'. Repeating this out loud several times will soften any unwanted emotions in these situations.

Most of us have made some bad decisions in life, but when we start to make the same mistake over and over, it's time to realise we need to find a better solution, to have a better outcome. We need to become more aware of where that 'little voice' in our head is coming from, and when it starts giving us 'reasons and excuses' why we can't do something we would enjoy, it's time to ignore its advice and find a way to do it anyway.

The annoying thing is, when we look back at opportunities lost by the Inner Abuser's reasons and excuses, we may also remember the little voice that came along after the opportunity had passed, telling us, 'maybe you should have just done that'! Yes, it's the same voice, it stopped you from enjoying the event, and then afterwards, suggested that maybe you should have just done it anyway. It gets two chances to upset you from the same event.

It created the 'reasons and excuses' to stop you from enjoying yourself, then after it was passed, created the 'regret' for not doing it.

The Inner Abuser gets stronger by feeding on the disappointment and regret it was responsible for creating. It's a cruel part of our mind, and one we must work on to control better in the future.

Start looking out for 'reasons and excuses' that self-sabotage your chances of a better life.

You might encounter something like this:

Authentic Self: 'I need to leave my partner, I can't take any more of his mental abuse.'

Inner Abuser; 'Yes, that would be good, but you can't leave just now, because ...'

- *'The house is in his name'*
- *'He controls all the money'*
- *'He would leave you penniless'*
- *'He will hound you until you go back to him'*
- *'He said he would kill himself if you leave him'*
- *'He said he would kill you if you leave him'*
- *'You have to stay until the kids are older'*

Fill in some of your own below ...

……………………………………………..

……………………………………………..

……………………………………………..

Superficially, all of these seem credible 'reasons and excuses', but in reality, a mental abuser's threats are just that, threats, but if your Inner Abuser is controlling your mind, it can create negative beliefs where the only thing you can imagine, is the worst possible outcome not the best. However, your belief is not necessarily the reality of any situation, and beliefs can be changed if we learn how to do it.

We have all been known to 'change our minds' throughout life, it's allowed, and it's healthy! It's also possible you may have a very different outlook in a few weeks, as you work with the exercises in this book.

Once you begin monitoring them, you can start to overcome the 'reasons and excuses' your Inner Abuser creates. Eventually, you can become skilled at dismissing them altogether.

₪

One of the biggest 'reasons or excuses' a woman can be sabotaged with, is thinking it's wrong to leave their abusive partner because the kids 'need' a father around. At first, it seems like a very legitimate 'reason' if you find yourself in this situation. However, this idea could be detrimental to the children's mental health. Children living in a home where they witness mental and emotional abuse on a daily basis can be affected by it. Negative influences can remain in the child's subconscious and affect them for the rest of their lives. The idea that kids need their dad around could be generated by the Inner Abuser to sabotage any thoughts of leaving. On deeper analysis the choice to stay with him can be a threat to your children's mental health and could scar them for life, depending on how severe the abuse they witness is.

Leaving him would mean he was forced into acting like a much more decent and reasonable person in front of them if he wanted to play any part in their future.

Many mentally abusive partners will create 'reasons and excuses' using the children as a bargaining tool to keep you and them with him. By realising that many of the 'reasons and excuses' you previously believed are not valid enough to control you any longer, you can eventually free yourself and your mind from his influence over much of your life.

Take some time now to examine 'reasons and excuses' you are holding as 'fact' and start to contemplate ways around them.

By repeating this regularly, you will empower your 'Authentic Self' and diminish the 'Inner Abuser's' influence from now on.

> *'How do you eat an elephant? ... in small bites'*

Every 'small bite' you take to regain control of your mind and so your life, empowers you.

As we already said, we all have an Inner Abuser. When we are further compromised by the conditioning of constant mental abuse, they both conspire against us.

The Inner Abuser is cunning, and that is why the 'reasons and excuses' it generates seem so legitimate, if they didn't appear so, they would be easier to ignore.

What we have to do, what we must do, is learn to recognise these 'reasons and excuses' for what they are, constraints made by our Inner Abuser to create more guilt, shame, stress and fear in our lives and ultimately keep us in an abusive relationship.

Try to recognise the 'reasons and excuses' that are created to sabotage your life, when they first appear. The more you do this, the easier it will be and the less power your Inner Abuser will have to undermine your thoughts.

This book is a new way to treat DMA, and the only way to realise it works is to follow the advice and the exercises. The traditional ways prescribed in the past, the ways that simply have not worked for so many women, and in many ways added to their suffering, are the alternatives on offer to you. When a woman tries to escape her DMA partner only to find herself, inexplicably returning to him and back under his control it has a demoralising effect on her. That's why it's so important to plan your departure properly the first time around, but only after mastering the exercises in this book.

A woman leaving her abusive partner and then returning, a day, a week or a year later is not a success at all.

Many women who manage to escape their abusive relationship physically, are permanently scarred emotionally, and this can hamper their ability to go on to have a joyful life and a loving relationship in the future. Just gaining physical freedom and not mental freedom is only a partial success. To help women to live and love again, learning from the past but not living in it, is why this book was created.

Every time you give in to 'reasons and excuses' that keep you in an abusive relationship, it would indicate your mind is not strong enough for the challenges of leaving … yet. Even if the belief that you cannot get away is buried in your subconscious right now, we can change it. We can dig it out and replace it with the belief that you can succeed in creating a new and better life for yourself.

When you become aware of any negative thoughts about your ability to leave to find a better life, do this little exercise:

Tell yourself out loud, not in thought (a thought alone does not have the power in it to help you), if you can't say it out loud, write it down, just thinking this will not have the desired effect;

'Stop right there!'

... and then ... even if it doesn't feel natural, do it anyway ... say ...

'I am going to succeed, I can have a better life away from him, I can do this'

Repeating this exercise often will help your subconscious rewrite the ideas it is holding at present. It will not happen overnight, but it **will** happen. Use it every time you catch yourself having negative 'reasons and excuses' that could sabotage your future happiness.

The power to choose your thoughts is in **your** mind, but when you give in to reasons and excuses generated by thoughts of your abusive partner, **you** are giving that power to him.

As you begin to understand more about the way DMA works, the way the Inner Abuser works, and the way reasons and excuses in your mind can sabotage you, you can also begin to take the ability to determine your own life back.

When you begin to realise that it is **your** mind that has been compromised and **it** has kept you in an abusive relationship, your abusive partner's hold over you will diminish. Believing your partner **took** the control of your situation creates the illusion that it is only he that can change it.

Soon, by understanding and strengthening your mind, you *will* be able to turn your back on your abusive partner successfully, leaving the future open to allow countless new opportunities to come into your life.

To succeed properly though, you must remain patient with this process a little longer.

Remember, the book will only work, if you work with the book. You cannot expect to get upstream if you float downstream. You need to start to swim.

These first few chapters are without doubt the most difficult part of the book to come to terms with, if you can do that, then you are well on your way to making a real difference in your life, using the exercises in Part 2.

Without an early explanation and your own understanding of the Inner Abuser's role in domestic mental abuse, the rest of the book would not deliver the results you are looking for. It had to come first. You have discovered the necessary elements on which to build the chance of a new life. Turning the attention on your Inner Abuser, and not your abusive partner will create the right mindset for you to recover and prosper after being manipulated by DMA.

The fight was never with your abusive partner and his attempt to control your life, but with the part of your mind that has aided and abetted him. It's a difficult thing to get your head around and for the moment at least, you don't need to spend too much time trying to understand it completely. At the moment the most important thing is to start working on yourself and stop focusing on your abusive partner's antics.

₪

The next chapter will help you decide which of the four categories mentioned before, best describes your present situation.

If you're still wondering about your own relationship, you could end up relieved if you find it doesn't contain any signs of domestic mental abuse after checking through the lists in the next chapter.

CHAPTER 4

RECOGNISING THE (HIDDEN) SIGNS OF DMA

Reading through this list may be disturbing for some. In particular, those that don't realise they are being mentally abused and specifically, those who are convinced they are NOT being mentally abused by their partner. It's a chapter that will be met with all kinds of emotion, sometimes relief and sometimes disbelief. Disregarding the emotional aspect of it, this chapter can also bring clarity to every woman that reads it. Try to keep an open mind while you contemplate the lists below, and remember, the truth sometimes hurts. When it comes to domestic mental abuse, it is better to discover the facts early, than to regret this opportunity and the chance to do something about it. Discovering some unpleasant truths now will work out better in the long run. To right a wrong, you have to know the wrong exists in the first place. Of course, in your case, it may not exist, so this information could help put your mind at rest too.

Noticing one or two of your partner's failings in this list will not instantly label him as an emotionally abusive man, but if you begin to tick more of the boxes, it's time to become more aware of the ones you haven't ticked too. Are you being completely truthful, or is your Inner Abuser trying to cover the truth up when you consider certain topics on this list? You may have to read this chapter a few times to consider more deeply each category below. As we have already discussed, if you are feeling you must rush through everything in your life, it could be a sign you are influenced by the effects of DMA and the Inner Abuser. If you find yourself skimming over this list, without giving each category due consideration, it's a possibility your Inner Abuser is trying to deny the truth, even if you are completely unaware of its influence.

Before you begin, remember that the second half of this book is designed to help you beat DMA and to assist you toward a new and happier life. Keep this in mind as you consider each example of mental abuse in this list. Even if you find yourself recognising a lot of these warning signs in your relationship try not to let this chapter overwhelm you. Remember we all need to know exactly what we are fighting before we can make a plan to beat it. Realising where you stand right now, is the first step to overcoming DMA.

After progressing through these lists, you decide you *are* being mentally abused, give yourself time to clear your mind, before contemplating your next move. Try to be truthful with yourself when considering each example. If your partner is using tactics that are not obvious signs of DMA, it can be a challenge to be honest with your answers. DMA is such a covert operation within a relationship, that it can be difficult to recognise, especially early on. Even when it becomes blatantly obvious to others, a woman can still, through no fault of her own, be oblivious to mental abuse even when it's right in front of her.

Consider the fact that this list is very important for your future. At this point, overlooking anything that indicates abuse may cause years of upset that could be avoided. You must give this your full attention, as it could be a pivotal moment in your life.

We can construct a list of traits associated with these individuals because they all use similar methods, similar phrases, and follow a similar course of action no matter where on earth they live. The global correlation in the methods of abuse they use allows us to recognise these individuals, predict their next move, and create an effective way to counteract and reverse the effects this type of abuse can have.

Firstly though, you need enough evidence to be convinced your partner is emotionally abusing you. Cognitive dissonance can blind you from believing what you see in front of you when the truth is just too difficult to accept. For the best results, go through this list slowly, contemplating each item in turn.

The internet has allowed women from all over the world to share their experiences on forums and social media, this can help them to understand how similar these experiences have been no matter where on earth they live.
Using the internet can also help women realise they are not alone.

This chapter covers other types of maltreatment too, like sexual and financial abuse as these can come under the umbrella of DMA. If you are unsure where you stand by the end of this chapter, look over it again with someone you can trust and confide in. Someone who is not influenced by your partner but may suspect he is not all he seems to be on the surface. (Remember, DMA camouflages its existence in your mind and you may need someone to help you uncover things your own mind just can't, or won't process at the moment. This is perfectly normal.)

One or two of these signs in your relationship doesn't mean you should automatically think about leaving your partner. Just be more vigilant from now on but don't discuss anything with him at this time. Monitoring the situation and looking out for the things you haven't ticked in this list should be enough action at this stage. Try not to become complacent, return to this checklist regularly to make sure he is not matching up to anything else here.
If you find yourself ticking five or more signs of abuse it is time to observe your relationship more closely. Be on your guard, while you read through the rest of this book and start using the mind-strengthening exercises in Part 2. Be careful not to create any suspicion in him, or show that your mindset has changed in any way. This is crucial for your long-term plans and your long-term safety.

Try to keep an open mind, just because you aren't entirely convinced he is emotionally abusing you, doesn't mean he isn't, it may be that you just don't realise it at this point … here is a very serious and necessary precaution on that matter:

COMPUTER, LAPTOP, SMARTPHONE OR TABLET, USE AND INTERNET SAFETY

Do not leave this situation to chance; from now on do not use your personal devices to surf the internet whilst researching DMA, or to send emails, texts or any other form of electronic messaging to discuss DMA with anyone else, whether it is a friend or a professional in this field. For that reason, this book is in paperback or electronic form, as long as you keep it concealed and don't purchase it using cashless payment there is no way of anyone knowing you are researching DMA unless you tell them. It's best your partner doesn't know you are reading this, at least for the time being. Some things are best not discussed at all and you are quite at liberty to read a book without discussing it with your partner even if you trust him implicitly. If you experience the urge to discuss the topic with him, it could be your Inner Abuser's influence, so sleep on it for a while, there is no rush and once you mention this book to him, there is no going back.

My advice would be this; even if you are convinced all is well after finishing this book, just move on and enjoy your relationship. You may find you have a renewed confidence in your partner and it enhances your relationship knowing he is not involved in a psychological plot to control your life. Arming yourself with the information here may allow you to assist others in the future. Reading it may be very worthwhile if you go on to help close friends or family avoid a life of pain and heartache, stuck in a DMA relationship. There is of course the added bonus that anyone using the exercises regularly will feel more alive and more in control of their own life.

॥

There is more information on the precautions of using modern technology later. Even if you leave an abusive partner, you may not be free from his surveillance. Monitoring mobile phones, emails or even bank accounts is common in DMA relationships. He may have surreptitiously gained the passwords or login details of any of your personal accounts.

Technology is now frequently used by mental abusers. It is never safe to continue using the same devices, numbers and passwords after discovering he is mentally abusing you. Make sure you take the precautions outlined later in this chapter (section 10).

It would make life a lot more difficult if you ignore this advice after being warned about it. Even more so, if you find out at a later date, that he has been monitoring you electronically, discovering your next move and using that knowledge against you.

I assure you this is one of the key areas you must be most vigilant, it is best to use a new cheap, talk and text phone on 'pay as you go' terms, the simplicity of these mobile phones makes them difficult to track. Smartphones are just too easy to keep tabs on. The same precautions apply to a tablet if you use it with a SIM card.

If you continue to research DMA on your existing smart gadgets because you are not convinced he is emotionally abusing you it could create unnecessary complications in the future. Especially if he does have access to your equipment. This is something you do not want to happen, so please take this seriously.

If you decide to do any research outside this book DO NOT use your own electronic devices or contact friends or relatives for their opinion through these devices.

DO NOT IGNORE THIS ADVICE AT THIS STAGE

₪

(You will need a pen to tick the boxes and underline anything you find below that relates to your situation)

COMMON SIGNS OF DMA

1. EMOTIONAL ABUSE IS A BIGGER PROBLEM THAN YOU THINK

When people think of domestic abuse, they often picture a woman who has been physically assaulted, but not all abusive relationships involve physical violence. Just because a woman doesn't look battered and bruised, it doesn't mean she is not being abused by her partner. Millions of women around the world suffer from emotional abuse in a relationship, and it is no less destructive than physical abuse. In fact, in many cases, it can take longer to heal and recover from.

Unfortunately, emotional abuse is often marginalised or overlooked – even if the person being abused doesn't recognise their partner's words and actions as mental or emotional abuse, they are likely to fob it off as a 'difficult relationship' rather than realise it is actually mental abuse. The shame of allowing the abuse to continue, or remaining in an abusive relationship can cause a woman to deny to others that any real problem exists. Sometimes those around her don't understand that mental abuse changes a woman's perception of her self-worth, that's why exposure to DMA needs to be better understood, and more openly discussed if we are to diminish its use in relationships overall.

2. UNDERSTANDING EMOTIONAL ABUSE

Understanding that the actions in the list below are mental abuse is important; they are not acceptable, warranted, part of a 'difficult marriage', excusable, or to be ignored if you want your life to be all it can be in the future.

Emotional abuse encompasses verbal abuse, shouting, threatening you, blaming you for everything and making you feel guilty or ashamed. Isolating you is also mental abuse. Additionally, emotional or psychological abusers often throw in threats of physical violence and other repercussions if you don't do what they want.

Because physical violence can put you in hospital and leave you bruised, battered or physically scarred you may think it's more serious than mental abuse, but the scars of emotional abuse are equally traumatic, although there is no sign of them with the naked eye. Many professionals believe emotional abuse takes longer to heal and is more difficult to fully recover from.

With emotional abuse, the insults, insinuations, criticism and accusations slowly eat away at your self-esteem until you become incapable of judging the situation objectively. You may begin to believe there is something wrong with you or fear you are losing your mind.

Or you may become so crushed that you blame yourself for the abuse.

DMA is a type of long-term brainwashing that will diminish your sense of identity, confidence and self-worth until you find yourself questioning your judgement and if you're being mentally abused at all.

DMA has many levels and these can differ depending on the dynamics of a relationship. Some abusers find it satisfactory to have a moderate level of control, and some want complete dominance over their partners.

Try to remember the old phrase, 'There is many a true word spoken in jest' while you make your way through the lists below. If he repetitively 'jokes' about something that puts you down, it's probably not a joke at all. So if you come across something sarcastic that he says in a jokey sense, consider ticking that box, or put a question mark beside it instead.

3. SIGNS YOU MAY BE IN AN ABUSIVE RELATIONSHIP

YOUR THOUGHTS AND FEELINGS, AND YOUR PARTNER'S ABUSIVE BEHAVIOUR
(Get a pen and tick the boxes in the list below that apply to you)

DO YOU:
- Feel scared of your partner on occasions? ☐
- Feel as if you are walking on eggshells? ☐
- Feel emotionally numb or helpless at any time? ☐
- Feel he is never happy with anything you do? ☐
- Sometimes think you deserve to be abused? ☐
- Avoid mentioning certain things out of fear of upsetting your partner? ☐
- Feel anxiety when he is due home? ☐
- Feel like you are on a daily emotional roller-coaster? ☐
- Think that you are the one that's unhinged? ☐
- Feel you are cut off a lot or even all the time? ☐
- Feel no one would believe your suspicions about DMA? ☐
- Feel trapped in the relationship? ☐
- Feel people will criticise you if you break up the relationship? ☐

DOES YOUR PARTNER:
- Humiliate you? ☐
- Yell at you? ☐
- Undermine your self-confidence? ☐

Domestic Mental Abuse

- Pick on things he knows upset you? ☐
- Guilt trip you? ☐
- Turn things around to make you the problem? ☐
- Never accept the blame? ☐
- Criticise you in general and put you down? ☐
- Make you feel embarrassed for your friends or family to see his abuse? ☐
- Belittle or ignore your opinions or abilities? ☐
- Blame you for his abusive behaviour? ☐
- Change the things he will and won't tolerate? ☐
- Put you down in front of your peers then say, 'I'm only kidding' or 'Don't take things so seriously'? ☐
- Does he treat you like a sex object or his property, instead of his partner? ☐
- Criticise your friends? ☐
- Criticise your clothes? ☐
- Criticise your cooking? ☐
- Criticise your job? ☐
- Criticise your intelligence? ☐
- Criticise your family? ☐
- Criticise your looks? ☐
- Criticise you in front of others? ☐
- Criticise your hobbies? ☐

Continue this list in the space below as you recall anything he has criticised you for that is not on this list.

4. YOUR PARTNER'S CONTROLLING BEHAVIOUR OR THREATS

DOES YOUR PARTNER:
- Have a bad or unpredictable temper? ☐
- Act excessively jealous or possessive? ☐
- Threaten to hurt or kill you? ☐
- Treat you like a child? ☐
- Block where you go or block what you do? ☐
- Threaten to harm your children or take them away from you? ☐
- Try to stop you from seeing family or friends? ☐
- Threaten to commit suicide if you leave? ☐
- Limit your access to money ☐, the phone ☐ or the car? ☐
- Force you to have sex? ☐
- Destroy your belongings? ☐
- Constantly check up on you? ☐
- Lie to you? ☐
- Lie to you when he is aware you know the truth? ☐
- Say, 'If you don't do this, I'll leave'? ☐
- Treat you with complete indifference? ☐
- Ignore or fail to answer your questions? ☐
- Leave the room if you ask a question he doesn't want to answer? ☐
- Fail to answer the question you asked, or answer a different one? ☐

Use the space to add to this list:

5. ABUSERS USE A VARIETY OF TACTICS TO MANIPULATE YOU AND EXERT THEIR POWER

- Dominance; Abusers need to feel in charge of the decisions in the relationship. They will order you to do things, and expect you to obey them completely, treat you like a child or a slave. ☐
- Humiliation; They will try to make you feel bad, guilty or unworthy. If they can make you feel unworthy, and unattractive to anyone else, you're less likely to leave. They will put you down in private and in front of others to erode your self-esteem. ☐
- Threats; They threaten their partner to stop them from escaping. He might say he will harm you or even threaten to kill you or your children. He may also threaten to commit suicide, or report you to the police making false allegations against you. ☐
- Isolation; To increase your dependence on him, an abusive partner will cut you off from the outside world. He might stop you from seeing friends, or forbid you from going to your work. He may make you ask his permission to go anywhere, or see anyone. ☐
- Intimidation; Your abuser may try to scare you by making threatening looks or gestures ☐, smashing things ☐ in front of you ☐, destroying property ☐, hurting your pets ☐ or putting weapons on display ☐. The underlying message is the threat of violence if you don't comply with his orders. ☐
- Denial and blame; Abusers are very good at making excuses for their inexcusable actions. They will blame their abusive and violent behaviour on a bad childhood ☐, a bad day ☐ and even on the ones they abuse ☐. He might deny

any abuse occurred or belittle it ☐. He will commonly shift the responsibility onto you, saying, his violent and abusive behaviour is your fault ☐.

Abusers can control their behaviour and they display this all the time.

- Abusers pick and choose whom to abuse. ☐
- They won't threaten or abuse everybody that annoys them. ☐
- They mostly abuse the people close to them, the ones they say they love. ☐
- Abusers carefully choose when and where to abuse. ☐
- They control themselves until no one else is about to see their abusive behaviour. ☐
- They may act like everything is fine in public ☐ ...
- ... but lash out instantly as soon as you're alone. ☐
- Abusers can stop their abusive behaviour when it benefits them. ☐
- Most abusers can choose their times to be abusive. They can stop any unsocial behaviour when it suits them ☐ (In front of the police, or their superiors at work for example).
- If DMA turns into physical violence, abusers usually direct their blows where they won't show. ☐
- Rather than acting in a mindless rage, many physically violent abusers carefully aim their kicks and punches where the bruises and marks are not seen by others. ☐
- Your abuser's apologies and loving gestures in between the episodes of mental, emotional or sexual abuse can make it feel more difficult to leave him. ☐
- He may make you believe that you are the only person who can help him ☐
- that things will be different this time ☐

- and that he truly loves you. ☐
- However, the dangers of staying with him are very real and abusers are masterful liars.

6. ECONOMIC OR FINANCIAL ABUSE IS CONSIDERED DMA IN A RELATIONSHIP

An abuser's goal is to control you, and he could use money to achieve this. Financial abuse can be:

- Putting the house mortgage in his name only. ☐
- Purchasing your car in his name giving 'reasons or excuses' to do so. ☐
- Purchasing your laptop, smartphone or tablet in his name. (This makes them easier to access or recover to investigate your private affairs). ☐
- Rigidly controlling your finances. ☐
- Withholding money or credit cards. ☐
- Making you account for every penny you spend. ☐
- Withholding basic necessities (food, medications, clothes, shelter). ☐
- Restricting you to an allowance. ☐
- Blocking you from choosing a career or taking a job. ☐
- Sabotaging your job (making you miss work, calling you constantly). ☐
- Stealing your money. ☐

Financial abuse can include not allowing you access to any money ☐, or putting you in charge of the budget ☐, but then spending all the money ☐ and blaming you when the debt mounts up ☐.

7. SEXUAL ABUSE IS A FORM OF MENTAL AND PHYSICAL ABUSE

- Any situation in which you are forced to participate or any degrading sexual activity is sexual abuse. ☐
- Forced sex, even by a spouse or intimate partner with whom you also have consensual sex, is an act of aggression and violence. ☐
- Sexual abuse includes pressurising you to have sex when you are sick. ☐
- Forcing you to have sex when you don't want it. ☐
- Forcing you to dress or act a certain way. ☐
- Forcing you to participate in group sex or use sexual 'toys'. ☐

People whose partners abuse them physically and sexually are at a higher risk of being injured or killed.

8. ABUSIVE BEHAVIOUR USED DELIBERATELY TO CONTROL YOU

- One-sided power games including behaviour that ensures he has his way at your expense. ☐
- Mind games including guilt trips and confusing you to make you feel depressed or mentally ill. ☐
- Inappropriate restrictions including refusing to let you work. ☐
- Isolation including controlling incoming information such as what you read or watch on TV. ☐
- Over-protection and 'caring' that includes dissuading you from going out alone in case you are attacked, raped, robbed or anything else that invokes the fear of being alone. ☐
- Emotional unkindness. ☐

- Violation of trust. ☐
- Cyberbullying, using electronic technology and devices. ☐
- Promising to help you and then 'forgetting'. ☐
- Degradation and suppression of your potential, including criticising your strengths and achievements. ☐
- Separation abuse including stalking such as leaving flowers – this sends a threatening message that he can always find you no matter where you are. (Don't mistake this for a 'caring gesture'.) ☐
- Using social institutions including engaging in child custody battles to maintain power over you. ☐
- Using social prejudices commenting on disabilities, or your skin colour and ethnic background and using them to empower himself. ☐
- Denying he is responsible for any upset. ☐
- Minimising the effects of his words or actions by saying 'It wasn't that bad, get over it.' ☐
- Blaming by twisting the story so you appear to be responsible for any incident or upset. ☐
- Making excuses for his words and actions such as blaming stress at his work. ☐
- Using children for example saying he wouldn't get so angry if you kept the children quiet. ☐
- Symbolic aggression including threats to harm family, friends or pets. ☐
- Domestic slavery including punishing you for not carrying out duties he claims you should have, while not carrying out his own. ☐
- Saying you bring out the worst in him. ☐

9. IT'S STILL MENTAL OR PHYSICAL ABUSE …

- … when any incidents of physical abuse have only occurred one or two times in the relationship. Studies indicate that if your spouse or partner has injured you once, it is likely he will continue to physically assault you in the near or distant future. ☐
- … when minor incidents of mental or physical abuse occur, compared to those you have seen on television, read about elsewhere or heard other women talk about. There isn't a 'better' or 'worse' form of mental or physical abuse. You can be severely injured as a result of him gesturing toward physical abuse. Even being pushed is a form of physical and mental abuse. ☐
- … when the abuse stopped after you became passive and gave up, your right to express yourself as you desire, your ability to move about freely, your choice to see others and to make your own decisions. It is not a victory if you have to give up your rights as a person and a partner in exchange for not being abused. ☐
- … when there has not been any physical violence. Many women are *emotionally* and *verbally* assaulted. This can be equally as frightening and is often more confusing to try to understand and recover from than physical abuse. ☐

10. THE USE OF MODERN TECHNOLOGY

One of the easiest ways to control a partner is to use modern technology and it is an area where many women don't recognise the dangers. It may be difficult to imagine your partner as an IT expert, but even the biggest technophobe can and will use technology to help in his control and his tactics of mental abuse.

Your partner may ...

- Constantly monitor your credit card use by having access to your accounts online (you may or may not be aware that he has the details, passwords etc. to these cards). He can check most credit card purchases on a minute-to-minute basis through the card provider's website. ☐
- Constantly monitor your debit card use in the same way. ☐
- Monitor where you are at all times by tracking your smartphone. This is frighteningly simple for anyone to do. ☐
- Install a secret app on your mobile phone allowing him to access all of the information on it remotely. These apps are invisible on the phone. He can take virtual control of all its functions; turn on the camera, take pictures, turn on the microphone and listen to any conversation it can pick up. He can also track the phone's position. ☐
- Many normal apps request permission to access; Body Sensors, Calendar, Camera, Contacts, Location, Microphone, Phone, SMS and more, but this spyware can do it without your consent. ☐
- Place a tracking device in your car, handbag, purse or even the hem of an item of clothing. These devices are very cheap to buy on the internet and can pinpoint your position to a few metres. They are small and difficult to find. ☐
- Install CCTV outside your home, claiming it's for security, but it is really to watch you, almost every CCTV system sold today can be accessed from a smartphone and watched 'live'. ☐
- Install CCTV inside the house and observe your intimate moments with him, or while you believe you are 'alone'. ☐
- Track your friends and family's phones just by having their phone numbers. He will do this to make sure you are really with the person you say you are meeting. ☐

- Retrieve all your personal contact numbers from your phone and record them. ☐
- Using his smartphone, photograph all of your documents, driving licence, passport, bank details, statements, etc. ☐
- Monitor your Facebook, Twitter, Instagram or other social media accounts. ☐
- Duplicate your email password and details and access them remotely at his leisure. ☐

I have witnessed every one of these techniques used to control and abuse women, even by abusers that appeared to have no technical knowledge. Don't think your partner is not capable of this type of abuse, it is best to believe he is and take the appropriate actions outlined later to prevent it.

11. HOW TO RECOGNISE THE SIGNS OF DOMESTIC ABUSE IN ANOTHER PERSON'S LIFE

It's impossible to know with certainty what goes on behind closed doors, but there are some tell-tale signs and symptoms of emotional abuse and domestic violence you can look out for in someone else's life.

If you witness any warning signs of abuse in a friend, family member, or co-worker, always take them seriously. If possible share your concerns with someone you trust and depending on the situation, the woman herself or the authorities. In every instance, you have to properly assess the situation for the safety of yourself and others before acting.

Women who are being mentally abused may ...
- Always seem anxious to please their partner. ☐
- Agree to almost everything their partner says or does. ☐
- Regularly call their partner to report what they're doing and where they are. ☐
- Receive frequent, harassing phone calls from their partner. ☐
- Talk about their partner's temper, jealousy or possessiveness. ☐

Women being isolated by their abuser will …
- Not be allowed to see family or friends. ☐
- Seldom be seen in public without their partner. ☐
- Have limited access to credit cards ☐, bank accounts or money ☐ or the car. ☐
- Get phone calls to come home early. ☐
- Get picked up unexpectedly early when out with others. ☐
- Cancel previously arranged meetings with others, even at the last minute. ☐
- Cancel engagements feigning sickness. ☐

The psychological warning signs of DMA in another woman may show as …
- Having very low self-esteem, even if she used to be confident. ☐
- Showing major personality changes (for example, an outgoing woman becomes withdrawn). ☐
- Signs of depression, anxiety or appearing suicidal. ☐
- Being very jumpy or nervous. ☐
- Getting agitated easily, or when her partner is due home from work. ☐
- Saying they believe their life is in danger. ☐
- Telling obvious lies, sometimes to cover up the abuse. ☐
- Take the side of her partner even when he abuses her in front of other people. ☐
- Telling others it's not that bad and that she can handle the situation with her DMA partner. ☐
- Leaving her abusive partner only to return time after time. ☐

After leaving their DMA partner, almost all women will experience some 'bad days', and they may start showing signs of remorse or pity towards him. (These are symptoms of the abuse they have been subjected to.)

Those around her have to accept that this will pass, but try to divert her attention away from this type of reminiscing. We can gently remind the woman, how truly awful the reality of that old relationship was. If given the right encouragement, this 'remorse' will pass quickly, and their resolve to beat these symptoms of DMA will return. Use the exercises in Part 2 of this book to become mentally stronger.

I remember one woman saying, 'That won't happen again, I will never want to go back there', and then after a few glasses of wine in a restaurant, she was saying she still loved her abusive 'ex' partner. She even talked about getting a taxi back to his house after the meal. Thankfully, she didn't act on the powerful influence her Inner Abuser was having on her at that moment in time. The next day she couldn't believe she had said all that 'out loud'. This is the long-term, preconditioning power mental or emotional abuse can have on a woman. It illustrates how our Inner Abuser can resurface at any time and try to convince us to do something disastrous to both our safety and our future. Overcoming those urges is part of the recovery process when working to reverse the effects DMA can have on any of us. As long as the abused woman does not remain in that mindset, no real harm is done as a result of a momentary lapse of reason.

These feelings of 'love' are residual, outdated thoughts that those affected by DMA can be prone to, especially if their mind is compromised by the use of alcohol or drugs which are best avoided altogether until their mental situation is stabilised. You will find more information on this later.

Although this book is primarily about beating mental abuse, signs of physical violence are included here as this can often follow mental abuse at some point in the future.

Women who are being physically abused may …

- Have frequent injuries, but say they were the result of 'accidents'.
- Frequently miss work, school or social occasions, without explanation.
- Wear clothes to hide cuts or bruises (e.g. wear long sleeves or trousers in the summer or sunglasses indoors).

If you suspect that a woman you know is being abused, speak up.

- If you're hesitating – telling yourself that it's none of your business, or think you might be wrong, or the woman might not want to talk about it – keep in mind that expressing your concern will let her know that you care and it may even save her life.
- Talk to the woman in private and let her know that you're concerned. Point out the things you've noticed that make you worried. Tell her you're happy to discuss it when she is ready. Reassure her that you'll keep whatever is said between the two of you, and let her know that you'll help in any way you can.
- Remember, abusers are very good at controlling and manipulating their partners. Women who have been emotionally abused are depressed, drained, scared, ashamed and confused. Women need help to get away from these men, especially if they have been isolated from their family and friends. By learning the tell-tale signs and offering assistance, you may save someone from an abusive situation.

FINALLY, TRY TO REMIND YOURSELF, MENTALLY ABUSIVE BEHAVIOUR IS THE ABUSER'S CHOICE

Domestic Mental Abuse

The mindset of a mentally abusive individual may stem from his genes and this personality disorder may have been with him since the day he was born. He may not have to plan the abuse, as it is natural to him, but the choice of whether he carries out the abuse is still something he can control. However, most of these individuals convince themselves they are in the right, whenever the abuse surfaces.

Despite what many people believe, domestic mental abuse is not due to the abuser's loss of control over his behaviour. He is choosing to manipulate you and your situation.

If you or someone you know may be experiencing DMA try to overcome any past or present emotional attachment to the abuser, and remind yourself he is choosing to treat you or a loved one in that manner. **You have to decide to change the situation because he never will.** Certainly not in a good way.

Often, mental abusers are committing multiple crimes.

In many countries, it is illegal to track someone on their mobile phone or with a tracker in their car or secreted in their clothes, without that person's knowledge or consent.

Forcing a woman to have sex even if you are married, is considered rape in many countries* around the world now. To force a woman into sexual intercourse if they do not want to participate is rape, even if she allows intercourse through fear.

Please check this with the authorities in your country before taking any action based on it.

Any financial abuse, withholding of funds, or access to money can be against the law in the country you live in.

Build up a list of the abuse you have been suffering and write it down, as you remember any instances from the past, or present, with dates and even times.

If the abuse was verbal, write down the words he used.

Remember, if he is creating any feelings of guilt or pity towards him in *your* mind, that is also considered mental abuse. For example, if he says 'It's your fault I did that' (said to create guilt in you), or 'I've been under so much stress at work and you don't care', (said to create pity and guilt in you). These are not random incidental comments, they are used to manipulate and confuse your thoughts, emotions and feelings.

Start recognising the words he uses to instigate a response from you. Think about the meaning behind what he says. Make note of his attempts to manipulate your mind when it happens, pay attention to 'why' he is saying it.

Begin to disassociate yourself from 'what' he is saying. Dispose of the words he uses and concentrate on **what he is trying to do to your mind** by using these words, or acting in a certain way: acting angry, huffy, in a threatening manner or seeking pity can all be forms of emotional abuse. Now and again we all have these emotions, but we don't use them continuously to manipulate our partner's thoughts.

Making a list of the abuse you have suffered is for your future protection. If you don't, you run the risk of confusing events and creating a lack of clarity on what was actually said and done. You are not breaking the law by making a list, ignore any inner feelings of guilt when you do this, **it is for your protection**.

Your partner is probably breaking the law by carrying out the things on your list. If you think his words or actions at any time could be considered DMA, but you aren't sure, include them anyway. There's a likelihood it will be, but you can remove them later if it turns out not to be the case.

Never feel guilty for trying to empower or respect yourself, that's what he wants. DMA is sometimes difficult to determine at first until you begin to study your situation in detail or retrospectively.

LIES

(A gentle reminder; have a pen or pencil handy every time you open this book. Particularly when you read it for the first time. It's easy to forget to do this but it is very important). <u>Underline</u> any sentences that particularly resonate with you and if you don't have one to hand please find a pen now.

I am going to ask you to underline this next paragraph in bold, even if you don't think you need to. It is so important you heed this particular advice. You may not get another free chance to do this correctly from now on.

Telling lies can cause all sorts of trouble to those suffering the effects of DMA. From now on try to resist the urge to tell lies, and in particular to those who are genuinely trying to help you.

If you are not honest when explaining your symptoms to a doctor, how can they diagnose the problem to help you find a solution? The same applies to those trying to help you diagnose a mental problem and help you escape a life of misery in a DMA relationship.

If you find yourself being questioned about your partner's abuse, but don't want to talk about it, try to resist the urge to lie, and instead of saying, 'I'm all right, he's not that bad', tell the person you find it difficult to discuss and will try to talk to them about it later … lies rarely make you feel better when you look back on any situation where you were less than truthful.

When you hear your abusive partner's frequent lies it desensitises you and creates the idea it is somehow normal to lie to people in your day-to-day life.

It isn't, and here is why …

You might not even realise you are being less than truthful when you try to take people's attention away from your abusive relationship. Saying things like 'He's not that bad', 'His bark's worse than his bite' or 'I can handle him' all seem easy ways to fend off other people's concerns, but is that really what you want to do? Is it not better to say you find it hard to talk about and that you might discuss it at a later date? If you deflect their attention or shut them down, you may just lose their much-needed support in the future. Think about it before you say something that just isn't true, from now on. Lying to those concerned about your welfare can have hidden consequences, you may not even be aware of.

There are many explanations an emotionally abused woman will give to cover up the truth of their relationship. I'd like you to think about how you have manipulated the truth to others recently. Before you do that, though, remind yourself that up until reading this book, you were unaware of your Inner Abuser, and therefore **IT** has been responsible for your previous misrepresentation of the truth. As we have said before, the Inner Abuser creates difficult situations and stress in your life any chance it gets. Misguiding those that are trying to help you may not work out in your favour in the long run.

Try not to feel guilty about any lies you have told in the past, you were not in control, and having any thoughts of guilt or shame will only serve to feed your Inner Abuser.

(*Without being aware of it you may have been acting under the influence of DMA and your Inner Abuser for some time now, so previous misdemeanours were made without your Authentic Self being aware of it. You are better to learn the lessons from past experiences and let them go than attach any guilt to them.*)

Now that you are using this book to help you understand what DMA does to a woman, it is best to make an effort to be truthful from this day on. Particularly to those around you that love and care for you. You may feel you have benefited from the little white lies you used to cover up what was happening in the past, but that is rarely the case. Many people will recognise even white lies and say nothing, but regulate their interaction with you as a result. Unfortunately from that point on they may find it hard to believe much of what you tell them in the future.

The use of lies to cover up his wrongdoing is another trick the Inner Abuser uses against you; for example, you can almost hear it say, *'Just tell a little white lie and you can get out of this situation, it's easy'* or ... *'Just lie to them, you can't deal with this right now.'*

At a later date, when you realise you have been caught, your Inner Abuser gets another chance to upset you by throwing this idea into your mind:

'Maybe you shouldn't have told that lie' or, *'maybe you shouldn't have handled it that way?'*

It loves creating guilt, shame and upset in your mind and it thrives on these emotions.

Take a moment to think about times you may have told a little lie to make things 'easy' and then lost that person's support because they knew fine and well it wasn't true.

Those who love and care for you may normally trust your word, however, if they discover you have lied to them in the past, it can be much more difficult to convince them when you eventually reveal the mental abuse you have been suffering.

You can, in many cases, redress this though, so don't allow your Inner Abuser to upset you by focusing on past misdemeanours. There is something you can do right now though, to reverse the harm that was caused by any lie you told in the past, no matter how small.

It is a small exercise, in the form of an affirmation.

This will help you in the future, take a deep breath and tell yourself out loud, right now …

'From now on I will not tell a lie.'

If you can't say it out loud where you are, use your pen and write it down here:

… and again here …

As we have said before, speaking out loud or writing things down is much more powerful than saying them to yourself. A thought does not affect your subconscious mind in the same way that listening to your voice speaking the words out loud does. Writing things down can have similar benefits if not quite the same powerful impact, even though you may not be aware of it at the time. The main thing is that you overcome the desire to ignore this exercise and do it, regardless of how effective you (or perhaps your Inner Abuser) believe it is.

This has been a little test for you; if you didn't say it out loud or write this down, you should try it now.

If you find this difficult or 'too much bother', this is a measure of how much influence the Inner Abuser has had on your subconscious without you realising it. If you chose not to participate in this affirmation, it could be an indication that your Inner Abuser doesn't want you to do anything to escape DMA.

Take control, show it you are determined to fight back against the influences it has had on you in the past and go back and do the affirmation exercise now.

You cannot beat DMA with this book, without following the recommendations in it. Even doing an exercise as small as this is an important part of reversing the changes DMA has had on you, without you realising it.

Please try to understand if you want to create a new life without DMA, you cannot do it by choosing what to participate in or ignore in this book. It doesn't work like that, and you will not reap the rewards if you don't follow these important steps in the manner described …

… let's continue, but only after the affirmation exercise is completed, don't let yourself down.

THINK 🠪 THINK

Think about gathering the courage to admit to those you can trust that you've not been completely truthful with them regarding your abusive relationship. You may get a pleasant surprise, confessing helps to destroy the lie and reaffirm with others the bond of trust you may have lost. Ask them to forgive and forget and to understand you have been under a lot of mental stress. It is advisable not to elaborate on your DMA situation unless you can trust the person 100 per cent. Remember, they may find it difficult to keep the information to themselves and may feel an inner (abuser) need to discuss it with someone else. The risk of opening up to them fully may not be in your best interest for the time being.

If you come clean over any small lies in the past but say you're not ready to discuss it further at the moment, that's usually enough to reconcile with anyone that cares for you. Give them time to process it and they will be by your side again, soon enough. There to help you with any difficulties you face while getting your life back on track.

It's worth reminding yourself how careful you must be with others, regarding any plans or decisions you forge for the future. The last thing you want is your abusive partner discovering them. Make sure you keep this book out of sight and think long and hard before you discuss plans with anyone. If your partner found out, he may become more abusive and controlling without necessarily telling you he knows of your plans. Keep any detailed arrangements to yourself, until you have read through this book and started using the exercises in Part 2.

From now on, being truthful with those you love and those you confide in, will help you achieve your objective. You will soon regain any trust you may have lost from friends and family that you were not previously completely honest with about your relationship.

Others being suspicious of you can come from your lack of honesty with them.
For people to trust you, *you* have to be truthful to them.
DMA and the Inner Abuser will try to convince you that lies make things easier, but their real objective is to see you push those who love and care for you away. From now on, be truthful, you'll be rewarded in ways you might not be aware of just yet.

If you are not still in a state of denial, and this chapter confirms your partner has been using mental abuse to manipulate your relationship, it will no doubt have come as a shock. Realising you have been living with DMA without being aware of it can be quite upsetting and the negative side of your mind, through the Inner Abuser may have you panicking and wondering what to do next.
If you are still processing it all, your mind needs time to adjust, and there are probably many questions you might be afraid to find the answers to. Accepting you have been deceived by your man can be deeply unnerving, but this acceptance has to be complete before you can then evaluate where you stand before making your next move.

It may help to think of the millions of women who have gone through life, lonely, isolated, confused, fearful and riddled with guilt and shame without realising all these emotions were a result of their partner's hidden mental abuse.

Right now though, confronting him is the last thing you want to do.

If you can recognise his abusive personality, you have the chance to do something about it. To ignore this information, will hamper your ability to overcome the effects DMA has already caused to your mind. To ignore this information will not stop him from continuing to abuse you either. As difficult as it may be, taking some time to process what you have discovered about your relationship is the best thing you could do. At the moment there will be times when you feel you can't even trust your own thoughts, many of which will still be generated by your Inner Abuser even though this chapter has been a big wake-up call.

Realise this is a pivotal moment and it can be a game-changer. Taking advice from others when your mind is confused by the situation, particularly those who have experience in dealing with DMA, is invaluable. Talk to someone involved with Women's Aid, or a similar charity, to gain some much-needed advice about your situation. By approaching people with expertise that are not emotionally involved, you can be more open without the chance of the information you share getting back to your partner, or others you would rather didn't know about your situation. At least for the time being. Remember, these organisations understand mental abuse much more than most and are not just there to help with physical abuse. Sometimes it can be better to confide in people you do not know. Your friends and family all have their own Inner Abuser, and it may well convince them it is acceptable to confide in a third party, possibly their partner ... but who might he tell?

When considering how to make a clean break successfully, it's better to keep any discussion distant from other family members who may want to get involved, and for your safety, it's best not to let them muddy the waters. Unless of course they have made it obvious they know what is going on in your relationship already. Discussing it with a counsellor at any women's charity will be in strict confidence and a way of getting it off your chest too.

Think about this. If by going through the lists above, you cannot ignore your partner's mental abuse any more, you now have some decisions to make. However, it would be wise not to make any hard and fast decisions right away. The realisation you are being mentally abused will still be very raw and this is not the time for knee-jerk reactions.

Whatever you do, do not confront your partner with any of the information you have discovered so far.

Seriously abusive men will be passive enough when you give them everything they want, abide by their rules, and succumb to their demands. If you can continue to put up with him for a little while longer, then it may be best to read this book through before you formulate a plan for your next move. Unless your situation is critical, or you absolutely feel strong enough to walk out the door, never to return, it is probably best to continue reading and do nothing to arouse suspicion at this time. If you strengthen your mind with the exercises coming up, your mind will soon be clearer, and any plans you make after that are much more likely to succeed.

If your mentally abusive partner finds out you are planning to leave or that you believe he is emotionally abusing you, he will probably change for the worse, overnight, and the tactics he might use to bring you back in line can be difficult to deal with for anyone.

Remember his biggest weapons are the things he says, and the way he says them to you. If you give him the chance, he will work on any guilt, shame or fear in your mind and use them all against you. His mind will only work in one way and that is to do or say anything he can, to convince you to stay in the relationship. He will use tears or threats in equal measure to achieve this. It will make no difference to him, as long as he gets what he wants. The fact is, he will do anything and say anything to get you to stay. In his subconscious mind, he owns you, and very few people like their possessions taken away from them.

For now, my advice would be to do nothing, and remember to keep this book in a place it cannot be found.

When you get to Part 2 in the book, start the course of daily mental exercises. Do them as instructed and your mind will become clearer, while at the same time, your Inner Abuser's influence will be diminished. After that, you will be in a much better place to make a plan for the future. You are not responsible for your abusive partner's future, you are responsible for *your own*. Make a point of reminding yourself of this from now on.

If you feel unsure about what you should do right now, do no more than continue reading. The more you learn the better equipped you will be to make the right decisions. Remember, the choices you make will impact those around you too, your children, your family, your friends and even your work colleagues. By working towards a clearer mind and better decisions, you will be helping all of them as well.

If you are slightly overwhelmed:
- You may feel you are not in a position to do anything about your situation at the moment.
- Or, convince yourself the abuse isn't too bad, in your case.
- Or, you might console yourself that he's not like that all the time and it might not be the worst life just to stay with him.

Even though it feels like your head is clear and you are thinking rationally, it could be an indication your Inner Abuser is controlling your thought processing. It could be masking your ability to consider your long-term future properly at this moment in time.

If you truly believe you are able to handle him at present, then try to think about your future. These individuals become more abusive as time passes and it would be sensible to give this due consideration if this list has revealed you are indeed living with a DMA partner.

In years to come, when you look back at all the heartbreak, fear, guilt and pain, hindsight will not be a comfort. The abuse may not be too bad at the moment but time will determine how controlling he becomes and how bad the future could be. This book is not designed to scare you into leaving your partner, but to encourage you to consider what your future could be like before deciding what to do next.

We only have one life, are you willing to dedicate yours to an abusive partner, who will probably get worse over time?

Is your mind telling you he isn't that bad because your Inner Abuser, fuelled by your partner's DMA, already has a grip on your ability to make decisions?

DMA is a form of long-term hypnosis, and most of us are not aware of any change in our mindset when it takes hold.

Years ago, when I was still researching, I came across one woman who was badly affected by DMA (I have yet to see worse), she was adamant she had not been brainwashed by her partner but knew he was abusive. She made many attempts to leave, gave up, and gave in to further emotional, sexual and financial abuse.

This book cannot help if you don't actively participate in your recovery from DMA yourself. That means, participating in **all** the exercises you find throughout these pages, and remembering to repeat them as often as you can. Repetition is the key, and you will find out why, later.

We have to take the responsibility to overcome these influences on our own shoulders. As daunting as it seems, when we talk about our minds, we are truly alone in there. Alone, with our black wolf and our white wolf.

It's a good time to decide which one you are going to feed, from now on.

It is imperative to consider what you have read up until now. Even if you have to start from the beginning again to grasp what DMA can do to your mind, your thought processes and the way you see the world.

No matter how good or bad you feel at this point … it is temporary. Nothing stays the same, especially our mood. It can get better or worse depending on what we feed it, if we want it to get better we must take control and feed that white wolf, pleasure, joy, compassion, gratitude and forgiveness.

By using this book, it is possible to change everything. With a little work and perseverance, you may soon be experiencing a different world, more positive and full of possibilities. Possibilities that are being denied to you at the present moment, as a result of past and present influences fuelled by DMA and your Inner Abuser. It is a road worth travelling if you want to live a fulfilled life and not just one dedicated to an individual that sees you as something he can abuse and control.

What direction will you choose, now that you know all this?

CHAPTER 5

UNDERSTANDING AN ABUSIVE PARTNER

I've heard many people say, 'I could never be taken in by mental abuse', however, DMA is so clandestine, that this particular belief leaves you more vulnerable to mental abuse, not less.

It is only learning the real facts about DMA that will prepare you for an emotional abuser's tactics.

You will only prepare a defence if you realise there is a danger, ignoring that danger will only leave you open to it, not prepared for it.

While reading this book, if you decide to leave your partner at some point in the future, please do not discuss that decision with anyone, especially him, until you have finished reading and more importantly, completely understand your situation and options.

Domestic mental abusers follow a similar pattern of abuse all over the world. They are born with an 'abusive gene'. Mental abuse can be predictable because these men follow this identical pattern. A pattern they were **all** born with, in the fabric of their being. If your partner is showing three or more indicators from the list of abuse in Chapter 4, he could be following the same template. Speak to anyone involved with the welfare of emotionally abused women and they will tell you many of the similar stories they hear regularly. Almost every story follows the same pattern, recreating the tell-tale behaviour of manipulation and control they all seem to use. There may be varying degrees of intensity, but the hallmarks of abuse are the same.

For those who understand the patterns they follow, this makes any abusive man's next move easier to predict. This isn't always apparent to an abused partner whose mind has already been affected by his mental abuse.

When you are in a relationship with an emotional abuser whether you feel it or not, your thought processes have been manipulated and compromised to some degree. How much, depends on how long the relationship has lasted and how intense his abuse has been. For the moment at least, try to consider if this is true in your case.

Regardless of what you discovered in Chapter 4, you may still think you could tell if you were being mentally abused or not, but it is unlikely you will 'feel' anything to help you do that.

It may be frustrating to think you are compromised mentally, but feel 'normal', and that's exactly why mental abuse is so successful at controlling people. You might have heard the phrase, 'love is blind', this could not be more true when it comes to DMA. The only difference is, that the emotion is not 'love', but an overwhelming feeling of attachment, installed in your mind over some time, by the words and actions of your partner.

Many women who are being emotionally abused cannot see it themselves, so in their minds, there is nothing to escape in the first place. They don't know that what's happening in their relationship is mental abuse. Yes, they hear the abusive language being used, they hear the threats, and it hurts emotionally at the time, but they are not aware of the long-term changes this abuse creates in their minds. They don't believe they have been 'brainwashed' and still want to believe that 'they are in control' of some aspects of their life. Even with the evidence in front of you, it's possible you still want to deny this could apply to you. That inability to recognise the reality of your situation is ironic, and a result of the mental abuse itself. Only once you accept your thoughts could have been compromised, can you start to do something about it. No one will fight an enemy if they don't believe it exists.

In between their abuse, these abusers can act perfectly normal, even 'loving' towards you, but this reverse psychology is just used to confuse your mind even further. This 'loving' side of him is just as abusive to your mind as the 'nasty' side of him. They are both used to grind you down and make you more compliant with his control. 'Good cop, bad cop'.

Many boxers continue in the sport even though they are aware of the long-term effect the pounding can have on their brain. Years later, they may suffer the consequences through an array of mental disorders caused by all those blows to the head. That's because each boxer believes 'I can handle it', 'I am different' or 'It won't happen to me'. Of course, it can, and in many cases, it does 'happen to them'. By ignoring the warnings, they are acting out the old saying, 'You're your own worst enemy'.

If someone warns you of danger, choosing to ignore their warning does not make the danger go away, it only means you will not be prepared for it when it happens!

It doesn't matter what you 'believe' is real, it only matters what **IS** real.

Convincing yourself that your partner isn't abusing you, won't stop the abuse, it merely blocks the idea of it and that will allow any abuse to continue, until one day you wake up and realise there is something wrong in your life but you feel too confused to realise what it is or what to do about it.

A woman may think she can 'handle' all the mental abuse thrown at her, but the long-term effects on her subconscious mind are real and devastating.

Understanding why an old boxer's hands are constantly shaking is relatively straightforward, but understanding why a woman continually leaves and returns to her abusive partner time after time, is not so obvious to most people. Few recognise this classic sign of long-term mental abuse, and many will just nod their heads and say, 'she needs a good shake'. Understanding the reason for many of the irrational choices a woman can make after years of mental abuse is not easy for a casual observer.

Discovering what causes **him** to be so abusive, will help **you** make better decisions. It will also help you understand that you cannot change him, and the only way to resolve **your** situation, is to begin to focus on yourself. He may say he will change, he may act out that 'change' for a little while (usually to convince you to stay with him) but he will not and sadly cannot, keep it up for long.

He was born with this personality disorder, it is in his genes and he cannot change and you cannot change him. If you mistakenly think you can, you may ruin your own life trying.

You may think you know best and *your* partner is somehow different from other mental abusers, but that is very unlikely. It may feel uncomfortable reading this, and you might want to believe you can change him, but sadly, what you want to believe and the reality of the situation could be two different things.

Mental abusers have an inborn need to dominate and control other people, but they usually concentrate most of their effort on their partners. Sometimes their children, their friends or their work colleagues can feel their wrath. Sometimes it can be members of their extended family, but usually, it is their partner or spouse who bears the brunt of their bad temper and mental manipulation.

- He may restrain his actions for a while if you confront him.
- He may promise not to repeat something that has upset you, but it won't be long before he does it again and blames you for it when he does. A common phrase used by abusers is, 'You bring out the worst in me'.
- He may agree to attend a marriage guidance counsellor but will take the first opportunity to stop you both from attending the appointments. He won't care that you see his reason for this as just an obvious excuse, because he simply doesn't care what you think.
- He may turn the blame on you, telling you it is your fault

for the way he is. (They use this a lot to create doubt in their partner's head, to lay doubt or even convince her, that somehow she may be to blame for the words coming out of his mouth.)
- He will not change because he cannot change; this 'abusive gene' is inborn, just like the gene for the colour of his eyes.

Even if you don't want to, once you accept you are being mentally abused, you have a decision to make. Will you stay with your abusive partner, while his abuse gets worse over the years, or will you use this book to help you avoid a lifetime of mental abuse? You do not need to make any decisions right now, continue reading, learn the facts and how to combat the manipulation of your mind that may have already taken place without you realising it.

If your head is still under your partner's influence, you're more likely to find 'reasons and excuses' why you should stay with him. Some of the reasons may seem very persuasive, but try to accept, at least for now, that it's very likely you are still under an abusive 'spell' … coupled with some help from your Inner Abuser.

Let's imagine David and Annie on their first date.

David seems to have a lot of the qualities Annie likes in a man.
They go out on a few dates and he seems pretty much ideal for her. His inborn abusive nature makes him do and say anything he thinks will please her. His subconscious will be following the 'abuser's blueprint'. By picking up the signs from her body language and their conversation, he uses the best ways to ingratiate himself with her. Meanwhile, Annie will have no idea he is being deceitful with this 'nice guy' act. It's worth noting that he is acting this naturally, he hasn't necessarily constructed a plan for it all.

Domestic Mental Abuse

She becomes more and more attracted to him and soon they move in together. By this point in time he's done and said a couple of things that she wasn't very pleased about, but all in all, he still seems pretty perfect for her. Her friends like him too, and he's popular in their circles.

Once his subconscious determines she has invested enough time and emotion into the relationship to make it difficult for her to justify leaving him, his mental abuse gets worse. Annie, still oblivious to his long-term abusive strategy, may think his demands are a bit annoying but not bad enough for her to leave him, and as time goes by she begins to capitulate to them. Any time she decides to refuse his demands, he will turn up the heat. Huffs, threats, guilt trips, shame, fear or even his tears will all be used to persuade her to do his bidding. By this time, if she dared rebel against one or two of his 'demands', she would experience the darker side of his nature. After learning the hard way, she will decide to go along with almost anything he demands, for an 'easy life'. She still thinks she loves him and uses that as the reason for the uncomfortable feeling of dependence she has on him.

More time passes (it could be years), and he eventually becomes bored of getting his way all the time and starts to make unreasonable demands on Annie. She refuses them and gets a barrage of insults and abuse ... it could be in the form of shouting or threatening violence or 'the silent treatment' or he might just disappear for a few days. The full array of his psychological 'arsenal' will surface to destroy her resistance and any of the willpower she has left. If one method of abuse doesn't work he will move on to the next. He might even buy her clothes, flowers or perfume to make her feel guilty about refusing his unreasonable demands, and she may naively think he still has a good side (without realising the only good side by then would be his back, as he walks out of the door). Annie may still be hanging on to the idea that she still 'loves' him.

Over the years, he may have decided, 'It's best to put the house in my name', and used a spurious 'reason' or 'excuse' to do so.

He might also have decided:
- *That he will 'take care' of their finances.*
- *He will decide where they go on holiday.*
- *She should do all the housework because he works hard and is tired at night.*
- *He will tell her what to wear, and constantly criticise her hair, her clothes, her friends, her intelligence, her family and what she cooks, eats, reads or says.*
- *If he is in a good mood, he will say these things as a sarcastic joke, if he is in a bad mood, he will say it with a threatening, noisy, intimidating snarl.*

His verbal abuse will become an almost constant, habitual presence in her life. By then she may just try to ignore it, but the abuse will continue to affect her subconscious and systematically diminish her entire self-worth.

This situation may take ten years, it doesn't matter to him and as long as it keeps going in the direction he wants, he may not have to become overly abusive. One day however all the pretence will end, he will be abusive on a regular and permanent basis and Annie will finally realise what she is dealing with but will likely be too weak mentally, to resist it.

There will be times when Annie thinks:
- 'He's not that bad'
- 'He's not abusive all the time'
- 'He has been nice in the past'
- 'He is good to others'
- 'It's a shame really, he is just sick in the head'.

These thoughts are just 'reasons and excuses' produced by her Inner Abuser, under the influence of all his DMA, to divert her mind from the grim realisation that he is emotionally abusing her and it is long past the time for her to walk out of the door.

Mental abuse will do that, it will make your life 'all about him' and not about you.

He may still try to appear charming in front of other people, but as the years pass, he'll find it increasingly difficult to keep up the pretence, and others may begin to notice his abuse. He may only drop his guard on the odd occasion, but if other people never challenge him, his abuse will become brazen in front of them, unless he is very self-controlled. (Sadly, even when they notice the abuse, it is common for other people not to get involved.)

Friends and relatives begin avoiding the couple more because the situation is too embarrassing, and it's easier just to stay away. They may even blame Annie for staying with David all these years. It's not easy when other people turn their back on your plight, but it's the easy way out for them, and in human nature, many people take the easiest route for themselves, not for others. Out of sight is out of mind. As a result of this Annie becomes more isolated from friends and relatives. If she tries to defend his abusive nature or lies to cover up the abuse, it may eventually turn the last of her friends and relatives away.

By this time Annie is a hollow shell of her former self and David blames her for all the things he believes are wrong in his life. Having a psychopathic nature, mentally abusive individuals are unable to see their faults and blame everything on everyone else, but most of all, on their partner.

If a mentally abusive man stood in front of a mirror looking for the person responsible for his problems, he wouldn't see his own reflection, but an image of his partner. These individuals are simply incapable of believing they are responsible for any wrongdoing. They will go to their grave with this belief. They may use words to say they are sorry and accept responsibility, but they don't mean it. Any apologies are insincere and usually designed to get them out of a hole or make them look reasonable when their wrongdoing has been exposed. This is just another form of mental abuse to confuse their partner.

The story of David and Annie is playing out in millions of relationships around the world, but few realise it, and those that do, are usually too ashamed to speak out about it. Many of the women that are being abused don't realise **it is** mental abuse, or they believe no one would listen to them if they were to air their fears, concerning their partner. Many friends and relatives witnessing this kind of situation are too embarrassed or scared to confront it, so they try to ignore it, or distance themselves from the person and problem altogether. These people are not to blame, but their inability to speak out about their concerns only helps to perpetuate abuse in our society today. The abusive gene passed down to these men has recognised this phenomenon in the human psyche, and adapted down through generations, to the abusive individual's advantage. By understanding how the human mind can be manipulated this abusive gene has developed the ability to use other people's human nature and psyche against them.

Using these generationally learned attributes against others' minds has worked so well in the past, that it has become part of the makeup of mental abusers. It's not just mentally abused people who have an Inner Abuser, we all do, and collectively, our society suffers as a result. This is why we all have a responsibility to recognise these abusers, and to work together to diminish their ability to manipulate other people's minds so effectively.

We must all play our part to eradicate DMA, and that is why all of us should learn how to strengthen our minds.

It is better to gain the strength to climb over the mountain than to sit down forever and wish it was not there.

SO WHAT MAKES A MENTALLY ABUSIVE MAN?

Almost everything I have researched about these individuals points to one thing …

He Was Born That Way and He Will Not Change His Ways

More accurately, it's not that he will not change it's that he *cannot* change. At least not for the better.

Just as he could not change the colour of his own eyes, he cannot change the nature of his own mind. He does not have the capacity to see the world as others do. He was born without the same level of compassion, empathy or understanding for other people's emotions that other human beings possess.

This may have been compounded by his childhood. Specifically, the years between two and twelve, but as a general rule, he acts like this because he was born like this. It is in his genes. He doesn't believe there is anything wrong with his personality, so he does not see any need to try to change it.

Your Inner Abuser may try to deny this is true for **your** partner, and recall some act of sympathy or compassion he has shown in the past to prove it. Remember, this Inner Abuser works against you and it may recall these 'acts of compassion' to discredit the facts being laid out in front of you just now. Try to keep an open mind and remember, these individuals are great actors. If they see a situation that they can exploit and ingratiate themselves with you or anyone else present at the time, they are quite capable of taking on the part of hero or saviour. By doing so, they deceive those observing and those that hear of the 'heroics' at a later date.

If you bring to mind a time when you remember him showing 'emotion', you may now understand he was creating an illusion to suit his ends. When these individuals act out a show of compassion they always gain something from it, and that could just be ... *your trust*. Could it be that his past 'illusions' worked and *that* is the reason you might still believe he has a heart? By previously creating the idea in your mind that he has some redeeming features, he also created a doubt that he may not be a mental abuser at all.

They are very persuasive individuals indeed, but remember, two wrongs don't make a right. If you ticked several signs of mental abuse in Chapter 4 and admitted he has abusive traits, you should not discount them just because you can recall some apparent acts of kindness he may once have committed.

Any show of compassion, empathy or sympathy towards others is generally insincere, even if it appears genuine at first sight. It's usually a move to gain credibility with those either observing it or those likely to hear about it later. He will take any opportunity to make himself look better in other people's eyes, even by feigning emotion where necessary. If he cries, it will be caused by his concern over the unobserved impact on him, not the impact on you or anyone else. As quickly as they can spout threats and abuse, these individuals can also turn on the tears at a moment's notice and especially if it aids in their quest to control other people's minds or perceptions. They don't need to think about it, tears will roll down their cheeks when their situation is in jeopardy, not yours.

He might cry because you have had an accident and broken your arm, but the real reason for the tears is that he will have to do the dishes or the housework, that's no joke.

He'll cry at a funeral to gain sympathy for himself from those around him, more than he is grieving the departed.

Remember his words are not to be trusted, they are designed to confuse your idea of him and also to mislead the people in the world around him.

At this point, your compassionate nature, backed by your Inner Abuser might be saying, 'Oh, come on, surely these people can show genuine emotion at a funeral?' I'm sorry, the emotion might be genuine, but not a lot of it is for the person in the casket.

If you're finding it hard to understand his lack of empathy, your Inner Abuser could be hampering your ability to accept it. This can be quite normal, particularly when you have always strived to see the good in everyone. Maybe taking a little time just now, to consider the difference between what you want to believe as opposed to what you are reading here. If you continue to be deceived by his 'crocodile tears' or when he helps an old person across the road, you are probably finding it difficult to come to terms with the boxes you ticked in Chapter 4 too.

Regardless of what he has managed to make you believe through years of DMA conditioning, in reality, he has very little compassion for others, and in particular, you. Certain facts are repeated many times throughout this book for a reason; to help the process needed to reverse the deceptive ideas he has been planting in your mind for a long time. One fact worthy of this repetition is that the ideas in your head may be a result of long-term DMA, and not based on the reality of a situation. It may sound strange, but just because a situation seems authentic to you, it still doesn't mean it is.

Emotionally abusive individuals are born with this personality, it is in their genes, and they cannot change.
They cannot quell their inborn desire to manipulate, dominate, control and abuse their partner. Just as 'a leopard cannot change its spots', an 'abusive individual cannot change his inborn and offensive 'nature'. They can hide it for brief periods, they can quell it for brief periods, but they can only appear to have changed it for brief periods too.

As a result of having little empathy or sympathy for others, they may not always be aware of how offensive their words and actions are at times. Other times, they are very aware of how cruel they are being and do it anyway. As a relationship goes on, many abusers get bored of all the attempts to appease them and bored of the submissive responses towards them. At this point, they may actively look for more and more cruel ways to make your life miserable, and many eventually turn to physical violence to achieve that.

You may not understand this at first but the best thing you can do to help him is to leave him …
… and the best thing you can do for yourself is to leave him. The best thing to do for your children, your family and the people who love you, is to leave him.

If you are the only target of his anger and abuse, once you remove yourself from the situation, he has no one there to focus his bad attitude on. If you're not around he has to mellow in the presence of others to appear reasonable or normal. Many abusers know this and temper their emotions to suit the situation, they also know if they inflict their wrath on others the way they did to their partner they'll lose any support, trust or confidence in them that they may otherwise have received.

He needs people to listen and believe him, to get them to participate in his plans to have you back on board. He'll probably try to blame you for the separation and cover up the real reasons for you leaving him. To achieve that, he needs to seem reasonable and honest to anyone willing to listen to him.

Meanwhile, you must be ready to repel those who get taken in by his lies. You need to be strong enough mentally, to resist being sidetracked by any rumours he may try to circulate. Stay focused on the single most important thing, your sole objective … that is, to get away from him and stay away from him. You probably know by now, if you have been subjected to a campaign of mental abuse that you were not previously aware of, the only way to find true love and happiness is to leave *him* behind.

The truth usually catches up with these abusers, when those around eventually realise what has been going on in your relationship. Most will soon see, if they haven't already, that his temperament is to blame for any separation.

Some patience and resolve are necessary, don't allow yourself to be drawn into any stories he tries to circulate, he will be hoping they get back to you for the sole purpose of upsetting you.

Abusive individuals and our Inner Abuser enjoy drama, be prepared for your partner to circulate his version of your break-up, and when it happens, simply try not to react. If there are people around you that decide to take his side, they may be people you are better off staying clear of, at least in the short term.

After you leave, if you don't talk to him, or allow him to communicate in any way; letters, emails, texts or messages through friends or relatives, you deny him the ability to abuse you any further, it's that simple. If he cannot get a message to you, he cannot abuse your mind any further. If you ignore all his attempts to contact you, no matter what avenue he tries to go down, he cannot manipulate your thoughts any more than he has. Of course, you will still have your Inner Abuser to deal with, but you won't have him to encourage it.

Remember:

HIS ABUSE COMES FROM HIS WORDS AND ACTIONS, STOP YOURSELF EXPERIENCING THAT AND YOU STOP ANY FURTHER ABUSE.

Abusers do know what they're doing, but as long as it looks like their partner is going to stick around and accept it, they won't temper their words or actions. While their partner continues to stay with them and doesn't complain too much, they don't believe what they are doing can be that bad. The fact their partner sticks around is an abuser's justification to others that his actions are not that objectionable. If their partner manages to make a good argument about the abuse, he might nod his head in agreement, but that's only to appease those present or to end the discussion.

In his mind, he has no intention of changing his ways … of course, that's mainly because he **can't**. He **can** temporarily stop, but before long his inborn need returns and so does his abusive nature.

If he manages to convince you to stay, he sees the capitulation as a weakness in you. He also sees it as a green light to continue abusing you. Maybe not right away, but soon after his hollow promises have had the desired effect and you either remained with him or you returned 'home' to him.

From time to time these men may appear to show some remorse, or tell you they recognise where they've gone wrong. This is usually just more deception and something else to mess with your head. As far as they are concerned they have a legitimate right to do whatever it takes to change your mind and get you back on their side. Any admission of guilt by them isn't genuine, and is another way of making you believe they won't do the same thing again … but they will.

They'll use threats or tears depending on the situation and won't care what anyone around thinks of them as long as they get their way in the end.

If you stay with him or return to him after he has made some hollow promises, it's only a matter of time before the abuse will start again … then after the next vicious outburst he might pretend to feel bad about it again, or he may blame you for inciting his abusive nature to resurface. Another tactic to unsettle you is to say you're being too sensitive. They will use whatever serves them best to mess with your mind, no matter what the situation. He won't need to sit and think about it either, his instinctive emotional abuse can find the most effective way possible to leave you feeling helpless and trapped.

Actions speak louder than words. He may **say** he will do this or that to pretend he is feeling guilt or remorse, but you will seldom see him fulfilling his promises to make things better for **you** in the relationship.

Abusers are masters at gaining your sympathy if they feel it will fulfil their agenda. Using sympathy against you though is just as manipulative as shouting, swearing or empty threats.

He will seek pity, play on your guilt, your shame, your fear or your love, it makes no difference to him. Whatever he has to do does not matter to him, as long as he regains control of your thoughts, he knows he can control your actions too. No matter what card he needs to play, he will, if it achieves his objective to continue controlling your life.

When it looks like you are going to leave, the biggest threat used by a domestic mental abuser, is, 'I'll kill myself if you go'. This is always done with great conviction and has convinced many women to remain under the same roof. Their Inner Abuser convinces them that his threat was real. In all the research I have carried out, it is extremely rare for this threat to become a reality. They know their partner's mind has been weakened by previous abuse, and as a result, are more likely to swallow this threat than someone who is not emotionally attached to the situation. Anyone with an understanding of how DMA works, will not be convinced by this overused threat, but a woman whose mind has been compromised by long-term mental abuse, is more likely to believe it, through no fault of her own. Now that you have reached this point in the book, you are more aware of the mind games these individuals play and are already less likely to be fooled by hollow threats.

If they choose to end their life, the responsibility would always remain with them and no blame could be accredited to an abused partner. The only accusations of blame would be from a woman's Inner Abuser, that's why it is so important to rebuild the strength of mind needed to deal with our Inner Abuser and these abusive individuals.

It is worth remembering that no one else is responsible for them, they are responsible for themselves. Try not to be swayed by threats of suicide, like so many other threats they make, they usually never dare to carry them out, regardless of how convincing they seem in the heat of the moment. These abusers rely on your fear, and you playing their game.

Imagine for a moment, one day, you just secretly left him, and imagine that after that moment, he could not communicate with you ever again. If that happened, there would be no way of a threat of 'suicide' ever reaching you. At that point by refusing to communicate you can safeguard yourself from any further abuse of your mind.

NO COMMUNICATION EQUALS NO FURTHER ABUSE

When I hear a woman saying, 'I couldn't live with myself if he committed suicide', I simply say, 'He won't, they never do'. Unfortunately, this 'suicide' threat usually stalls a woman when she is on the verge of leaving and it's why these abusers all use it. If you end up in that situation and feel the need to give in to it, your mind may still be heavily influenced by the damage from past DMA. Using the techniques in this book will help you see his threats in a different light in the future.

'I'll kill myself if …', is one of the most common guilt trips an abuser will use to bring their partner back into line and make her afraid to leave in the future.

He will use fear more than anything else to try to control you.

Maybe you should underline that sentence with your pen or highlight it on your electronic device.

- In mental abuse, his best weapon is **the idea** that he will do something rather than him doing it, remember mental abuse is an attack on the mind, not the body.
- He will try to incite pity **for** him, or fear **of** him.
- He does not care, as long as he gets what he wants … and what he wants is for you to capitulate to his will, wishes or demands.
- He doesn't care how pathetic he looks, or how crazy he looks to anyone else either, what other people think does not matter to him, as long as he gets what he wants.

He will feign any emotion to you and others, he'll break down and cry real tears for hours on end if he thinks it will achieve what he wants. A woman told me her abusive husband cried all night to get her to come back to him, and promised time after time, through his snivelling, that he would change his ways. She capitulated and moved back into their home, whereupon just a few weeks after she had returned to him, he began a regime of sexual abuse culminating in rape, and after that, she told me, it became a regular occurrence.

He would sit at the breakfast table the next morning and apologise for his actions of the previous night, saying it would never happen again, but she told me, it did. Please underline this short but tragic story, and remember, in the case of mental abusers, falling for his promises or lies can have dire consequences after you capitulate.

The punishment for daring to disobey him is not always sexual or physical abuse, but they will often increase their mind games to break your spirit completely.

When his abuse is witnessed by someone else, he might apologise to you, in an attempt to minimise any repercussions others may feel compelled to initiate, like informing your family or even the authorities. He may also take a break from abusing you if he thinks there may be any consequences from others observing his abuse, but after a short time and once the memory of the incident fades, the abuse will resume.

Usually, they have no empathy, they are not born with it and they cannot gain it or manufacture it within themselves, they are simply not capable of that.

It is worth repeating the point here, it's important to be very careful, if you believe your partner is incapable of escalating his verbal insults, to sexual or physical abuse. Underestimating him can be very costly indeed.

Some of them, usually younger men, may try to take control too soon and lose partners due to a lack of finesse in their crude attempts to manipulate the relationship. They learn from these mistakes though and become more adept at handling future partners' thoughts, using the knowledge they gained from the previous relationships.

Finally, since we are talking about mental abusers and not physical abusers here are some of the things they will do to mess with your mind and grind you down.

They don't use their physical strength to lock you up or beat you into submission. The biggest weapon is their words … **Mind games.**

The ability to control someone else just with words sounds too good to be true, too simple, doesn't it? Yet that is exactly what mental abusers do. Sometimes they might raise their hand but in the early days at least, they are usually feigning and will not use physical violence.

Whatever they do or say, their use of fear tactics is usually never far away. Fear is a great way of gaining control over people's minds, it has been used for thousands of years and is extremely effective. Much of what an abusive partner says is designed to promote fear in some form, control your mind and change the way you see the world.

From now on, try to notice the effect his words have on you, and how you feel physically as well as emotionally. Try to monitor your thoughts when he is being abusive towards you, and remind yourself what he is trying to do to your mind.

Look out for the trigger words and phrases he uses and repeats to upset you.

Notice how they make you feel, does your chest tighten, your stomach flip or cramp? Do you have a 'brain freeze', when you find it difficult to think clearly? He says things to invoke a certain reaction in your mind. Then your thoughts create an emotion, and the emotion, in turn, creates a physical feeling. Just by using certain keywords or expressions, he can cause a fearful reaction in your mind and create certain feelings in your physical body as well. This is the power his words can have. You don't need to be involved with mental abuse to be affected by someone else's words. Words are powerful, and the way they are delivered is powerful too.

Although his mind games are only as effective as you allow them to be, the longer you are subjected to mental abuse, the more difficult it is to realise where a normal conversation with him ends and his words designed to manipulate your thoughts begin.

This is why it is important to strengthen your mind, before making a proper plan for your future. Soon, you will begin working with the exercises that will help you do that.

Domestic Mental Abuse

People have been well aware that we can use words to control others' minds for a very long time. The word 'spelling' was first used in England in the Middle Ages. It is based on the word 'spell'.

The dictionary gives these descriptions of the word spell:

- *A word, phrase, or form of words supposed to have magic power; charm; incantation: The wizard casts a spell.*
- *A state or period of enchantment: She was under a spell.*
- *Any dominating or irresistible influence.*

The early use of the word 'spelling' almost a thousand years ago, is proof that people realised how effective using the right words (spelled out) and phrases or sayings could be to control the thoughts, emotions and feelings of others, and of the masses. By understanding this timescale, we know that mental abuse has been used and handed down through generations, for at least a thousand years.

Today those that use this knowledge to control their partners are known as domestic mental abusers or emotional abusers. They are the descendants of the manipulative individuals from long before the Middle Ages that realised words could cast spells and spells can cause fear. If we had no fear, we would not be as easily manipulated.

Fear can present itself in many ways, once it is installed in our subconscious it can take hold of us and consume much of our lives.

Look out for this, and consider what the real reason is for a sudden rush of fear. Has your partner conditioned a fearful mindset in you?
Are there subjects you know not to talk about?
Are there people you know not to see?
Are there places you know not to go to?

I hope you are beginning to realise that trying to get a return to those days with 'the guy you first met' is not an option. 'That guy' was most likely a disguise, an act and a con. A facade, he naturally created, without much conscious planning, to steal your heart and your mind, and to control you at a later date. You cannot get the 'original guy' back because he never truly existed and you could waste the rest of your life attempting to resurrect the 'dead'.

I know that may seem harsh, but until you surrender to this fact, your life may continue to be a struggle much of the time.

One day, you may find a man that will treat you with love and respect, but it will not be this man.

Something to keep in mind about an emotionally abusive partner …
He will not change … he will not 'get better' … and believing you can change him, will still change nothing.

In part, he created that very idea in your head to control you, he created the idea that you can somehow get 'that old guy back'. He acted the part of the perfect partner when you first met, for this very reason. Who wouldn't want to resurrect their perfect partner from the ashes of the mental abuser they find themselves with?

Don't be fooled. Once they show their true character, they simply can't be bothered to keep up the act any longer. They don't need to, because, in their eyes, you have reached the point where they do not envisage you ever having the courage to leave.

All you can do is recognise and accept that the 'perfect partner' never existed in the first place and therefore, you cannot get him back. It was only an illusion he created to trap you … forever.

The sooner you can accept that he will not change for the better, the sooner you can begin to reverse the effects of his mental abuse.

You would need to be lottery-winning lucky to change him, sadly though, too many women have wasted their lives believing they could. This part of his personality is hard-wired into his being, he will not change and all the research supports this.

There is a part of us all that would like to show a mentally abusive individual the error of his ways, in the hope he could become a better person, but we would fail in the trying.

Their minds are simply incapable of understanding they should change the way they act, and anything negative that happens between you both is your fault, not his.

Your Inner Abuser will try to convince you time after time, that 'this time', he'll change. He won't and until you recognise this is a trap created by both, his 'spell' and your Inner Abuser, you will continue to waste precious time trying.

Mental abusers are not the right choice for any chance of a happy and contented future. If you ticked a lot of the boxes in Chapter 4, you already know his true character. The challenge now is to be able to accept it and only then can you begin the process to reverse the effect his abuse has had on your mind.

A final word on him ...
It's not like he sits at night and plans how he is going to condition your mind the following day, most of this mental abuse comes naturally to him, moment by moment. Much of it comes from his subconscious and he acts the part without any effort. As the relationship continues and he gets bored of the dominance he created, he may then actively engage his mind to start dreaming up new ways to abuse and control you even more. If you try to leave him, he will escalate his abuse substantially, making it more difficult for you to escape in the future. In some cases, he will take pleasure in plotting how to upset you, unsettle you, make you jealous, make you feel guilty or make you worried, scared or fearful.

There are many things to come to terms with when you discover you are in an emotionally abusive relationship, it may help you to repeat this mantra when you feel yourself feeling compassion for the plight he has created for himself:

HE IS A MENTAL ABUSER, HE WILL NOT CHANGE
HE IS A MENTAL ABUSER, HE WILL NOT CHANGE

HE won't change for the better
YOU will never change him for the better
HE will get worse over time

HE IS A MENTAL ABUSER, HE WILL NOT CHANGE

₪

This isn't an easy lesson to learn, and accept. By doing that, it doesn't mean you have lost anything, on the contrary, you have gained the knowledge needed to start making a much better life for yourself. Even if it doesn't feel like it, that's a good thing, right?

Now you know you can't change **him** and you know if you want to change **anything**, you must begin to change **yourself**. This is where the power you lost was hidden; the idea that you were powerless to change anything. You are not powerless you always had the power in you to change, you just misplaced the knowledge in your mind that you are capable and strong enough to overcome the effects of a mental assault like this. From now on, it is your responsibility to stop the Inner Abuser from sabotaging your efforts to change your life.

Accepting this idea ...
'If you want change, it is you that needs to change'
... is when you begin to take back control.

- You can start planning to leave him (if it's not for the first time make it the last).
- You no longer need to consider him (he can do that for himself).
- You no longer need to consider his 'feelings'.
- You no longer need to consider how happy he is.
- You no longer need to consider keeping him happy for the rest of your life.

These all become his responsibility to himself, not yours.

Start considering yourself and your happiness. If that means continuing to act as the same submissive partner for a while, then at least you can reassure yourself it is not forever, but simply to help come to terms with your new power, and to strengthen your mind. When considering the facts that surround mental abuse, it is difficult to leave successfully without a plan, and without strengthening your mind enough to deal with his manipulative personality, even after you have left him.

Even if you make a plan, a good plan, your chances of success are weakened if you do not first use the exercises in this book, to strengthen your mind, your will and your resolve.

Your mind has been affected by his constant repetition of mental abuse for a long time. By constant repetition of these exercises, you can reverse the changes caused by that abuse.

- **Any time you find yourself considering his thoughts and feelings, immediately ask yourself why you are not considering your own instead?**
- **Do this every time he enters your head.**
- **You can only have one thought in your head at a time, make a decision right now, never put thoughts of his 'feelings' ahead of yours.**

It will take time to master this exercise, and you have to accept, that at first, he will continue to dominate a lot of your thoughts. That is okay. You are human, and that is the way the human mind works. So, if he comes into your head a hundred times a day, as soon as you notice that your thoughts are considering him, you change them, even if it actually is a hundred times a day, to begin with.

As the days go by, you will get better at this, you will begin to notice he is not appearing in your mind quite so much and you will start to realise a change is taking place.

₪

Although he was born this way, he is aware of what he is doing, he can turn it on and off when he wants, and he consciously and subconsciously chooses the timing of his abusive words and actions.
It is fundamental to your recovery to remember this …

HIS GREATEST WEAPONS ARE HIS WORDS

₪

He may say them out loud or write them in an email, text or social media message or ask a third party to relay a message to you. It doesn't matter how he tries to get you to listen to his words, it is still a direct attempt to use his greatest weapon to control your mind. Always try to remember this.
I want you to think about this for a minute or two …

- **WORDS** are his biggest weapons.
- He uses **WORDS** to manipulate your thoughts, emotions, and feelings.
- If you stop his **WORDS** from reaching you, you stop any further abuse from reaching you.

- If you take away his **WORDS** he can't do any more damage to your mind ...
- ... and then your mind can start to recover from the damage already done.

(To take away his words completely, you have to make sure he cannot contact you, and the guidelines to help you achieve this are described later.)

So how do you take away his words?
Strengthen your mind by using this book regularly. This will help reprogramme the way you think and enable you to undo the damage his long-term abuse has caused to your thought processing. The only way you are going to discover how well this works is by doing these exercises yourself. You cannot predict how this will help you, you cannot listen to another individual's opinion because they cannot predict the outcome accurately either ... you have to do the exercises yourself to find out how effective they are for **you**. There is no short cut I'm afraid.

Anyone, regardless of their profession, who questions the transformation these exercises can have for someone suffering from the effects of DMA, has never used them properly for themselves.
You will never fully understand a lost opportunity if you do not experience it in the first place.

There are millions of men who use milder forms of mental abuse to gain a certain amount of control in their relationships and remain content once they achieve the level they are comfortable with. Most of the time their abuse is tempered by your submission to a lot of their demands. They may allow you to feel you have some choices, as long as they know they can take control any time they want. It may not be obvious to you, and you may feel you have some freedom, but these will only be things he is not concerned about controlling. In his mind, he is allowing you **some** 'freedom', to create the illusion you have **complete** 'freedom'. It's a gilded cage, and he has the key. A time may come when he wants to take more control of your life than he has at the moment.

These abusers elevate themselves to whatever level of control they want, then back off, even if you don't notice this happening. If you step out of line they know they have the power to remove the 'freedoms' they have 'given' you, any time they like.

If you dare to threaten their control along the way, you will soon discover a very different individual.

CHAPTER 6

IF YOU WANT TO OVERCOME DMA ... YOU ... NEED TO CHANGE
ACCEPTING THIS, MARKS THE BEGINNING OF YOUR RECOVERY

Think of it this way, the previous chapter explained why we cannot change the mind of a mental abuser, so if you want anything to change in a DMA relationship, accepting the only way forward is to change your own mind opens a future full of possibilities.

What can I change about myself?
My mind? Change my old mind, my old limiting beliefs, for some new non-limiting beliefs?

But maybe, you might be asking yourself, why should 'I' change, and not him?

The answer is this; if you are unhappy about your present situation, then the part of your mind that made the choices to get you into the present situation has not served you well. We can call that part of your mind, the 'old you'. So, if you're not happy with things right now, it makes sense not to allow the 'old you' to make any more decisions, or you can expect much of the same results. If you have a DMA partner, the chances are, the 'old you' guided you into that relationship too and has been making all the decisions that have kept you in it.

The main reason the 'old you' brought you to this moment in life is your Inner Abuser, and we know it creates drama and upset whenever it can.
So, if the 'old you' was responsible for all the bad decisions that got you into your present predicament, then you don't want to let the 'old

you' make any more decisions, do you? Hopefully, the answer is 'no', and that means we have to create a 'new you'.
How do you do this?

First ...
If you didn't follow the doctor's advice, can you expect to recover from an illness?

If you don't get better, can you blame the doctor?

₪

The same applies to this book, if you didn't follow the advice, can you expect to recover from DMA?

If you don't follow the advice and your life doesn't get better, can you blame this book?

DMA is serious, so the advice to beat it must be taken seriously too.

Now that you are aware it exists, your Inner Abuser and its negative influence should become more obvious to you, as you begin to observe your thoughts more often. Be vigilant of its attempts to stop you working with this book.

The battle is in your mind, like the story of the two wolves, starve the Black Wolf, Inner Abuser, 'old you', and feed the White Wolf, Authentic Self, 'new you'.

As you become more interactive with this book, the 'new you' will learn how to make better decisions, stay positive and keep learning ...

The Inner Abuser will try to convince you there are recommendations in this book that in your case, *can be ignored*. Be careful, everything you are asked to do regarding the improvement of your mind is here for a reason. Each exercise tweaks your thought processes in slightly different ways. You DO need to use them ALL.

Remind yourself …
- I want to beat DMA completely.
- My Authentic Self wants to beat DMA completely.
- My future self wants to beat DMA completely.
- I need to put a little effort in for this to happen.

Follow these guidelines, and ignore your Inner Abuser when it pops up to question or criticise them. How much you change should be the choice of your new Authentic Self, not the 'old you'.

Recognising what part of your mind is making the choices can be challenging to begin with so don't get upset if you find you are slipping into old thought patterns. When you notice them returning (you will), just reset your thoughts and reaffirm your intention to make sure your decisions are coming from the 'new you'.

After reading the last chapter you know you cannot change your abusive partner, therefore the only way to make a positive difference in your life is to change yourself.

The power to make positive changes comes from within, if you expect others to change things for you, you are giving that power away, and much of the time, to your abusive partner.

**If nothing changes, it remains the same, and that is not what you want.
To change your life you have to change your mind.**

You must *really* want to change and this quick exercise will help to begin the process …

Sit down, get relaxed and take a few deep breaths, then, once you're ready, say out loud …

'I WANT TO CHANGE, I WANT THIS'

… repeat it out loud at least ten times, or, if you're in a place where you cannot speak, make sure you write it down ten times. Feel it inside you, and mean it when you say it.

As before, just thinking it is not powerful enough and you will gain very little from this exercise if you don't say it out loud, or write it down.

This is very important because the more you say or write 'I WANT TO CHANGE, I WANT THIS', the more your subconscious will realise it has to start finding ways to make this change happen.

The 'old you' and your Inner Abuser have been making a lot of bad decisions that have brought you to the situation you are in now. Changes have to be made to stop more bad decisions. Reducing its ability to control your thoughts will allow your 'Authentic Self' to become stronger, take control and make better decisions for the 'new you', from now on.

If you commit to changing yourself, it can be a defining time in your life, even if you don't fully understand that yet.

Every time you use this simple affirmation, 'I WANT THIS, I WANT TO CHANGE', positive ideas will begin to surface in your mind. Repeating it will make a big difference to your subconscious. It is called your subconscious or your unconscious for that reason, we are not openly aware of the changes happening at that level. Look out for your Inner Abuser telling you all this won't work, and every time you recognise it trying to manipulate your thoughts, dismiss it. This affirmation works, all you need to do is repeat it regularly throughout the day. The more you say it, the more real that change will become.

If you can't say it out loud, write it down on a new piece of paper. You *cannot* read over the piece of paper you wrote it on the last time.

That does not help to reprogramme the subconscious.

If you want something amazing to happen on the inside, then keep telling yourself on the outside …

'I WANT THIS, I WANT CHANGE'

… and mean it.

₪

If you ever thought of yourself as a victim, try to understand, that you were only a victim of your Inner Abuser because you were unaware of its existence. You believed your thoughts were being generated by you, or what we know as your 'Authentic Self', and therefore expected those thoughts to be for your own best interest.

Those ideas you had in the past, were not created for an easy life, they were created for a difficult one. By being more aware of your Inner Abuser, you can reduce the number of unhelpful thoughts you have from now on.

You may have been convinced you were trapped in a DMA relationship and couldn't do anything about it. Now, by using the affirmation above, your subconscious will produce new and better ways to look at your situation and find a safe way out of it.

The old version of you succumbed to DMA, the new version of you will reverse the effects that DMA had on you.

How quickly it happens depends on how hard you work with all of these exercises.

Repetition is the key, the changes will follow and make themselves obvious in time. Your mind will start to generate new unique ideas to deal with your situation. Your life will transform as you begin to feel stronger mentally, implement changes and start to benefit from them.

One of the changes to make is to stop overthinking.

₪

OVERTHINKING

To understand the influence our Inner Abuser has on our thoughts, it's helpful to become aware of something that causes many of us unnecessary anxiety in our lives, and we don't even realise we are doing it. It is called overthinking, and it is also the source of so much unhappiness in the world.

No one teaches us how to recognise when we are overthinking and more importantly we are not taught what we can do to stop it.

We are not taught how to use our brains to benefit our own lives the most. What we think about is literally the world we create for ourselves in our minds. If we are always thinking of the past, possibly the bad things that have happened to us, or regrets we have over things we did or didn't do, we are literally living in the past at that moment. If we are living in the past at that moment, we cannot be living in the present, at least, our minds are not in the present.

Equally, if we worry about the future, that is, things that haven't happened yet (and may never happen) we are not living in the present either.

We miss out on the actual reality of our present situation.

About now, your Inner Abuser will be doing its best to discredit this idea, but keep an open mind and read on ...

Overthinking can cause anxiety, stress, insomnia and lead to depression. Much of the overthinking we do is described by one word ... worry. We worry too much.

In many cases overthinking is like an addiction, and one way to overcome it is to practise focusing on the present moment. This, of course, like many of the exercises in this book, sounds easy but takes a bit of time to perfect. However, with practice and repetition, it is possible. When you master it, this can truly be life-changing. If it was easy, we would all be doing it already. Learning to focus on the present stops us from fretting over the past and stops us from worrying over the future. This exercise is just simply **remembering** to bring yourself back to the present moment every time you find you have wandered off into unhelpful thoughts of the past or the future.

The only things a trained mind will take from the past are the lessons it taught us, the only things a trained mind will consider in the future, are necessary plans for the days ahead, without worrying about them. Anything else is unnecessary. This might seem harsh, but if you practise adhering to these recommendations, you will have much more time to take in what you are doing right now. If our mind defaults to living in the past or the future, it cannot be as aware of the present. When this happens we miss the richness of the moment we are in. We are actually missing out on life as it happens in real time.

Make it a habit to check in on your thoughts and then *stay* focused on what is happening in the present moment and immerse yourself in it, whatever you are doing and wherever you are.

₪

Did you notice the sign above that means you should stop and think about this?

The reason I ask, is that at this point in the book, making the decision to 'stop and think' about what you have just read is important. Reminding yourself to 'stop' and to 'think' about your thoughts, is the key to observing those thoughts, and adjusting them as you go through the day.

For example; as your mind drifts from subject to subject, practise becoming aware of each subject as it enters your head, you can then decide if it's necessary to think about that 'subject' at that time. You can also ask yourself, 'Is this thought making me feel bad, or good?' and 'Is this thought serving me well?'

'Do I need to think about this right now?' is a good question to ask yourself. It can dissolve anything from the past or future that is stealing your joy but does not need to be addressed at that time.

If your answer to that question is, 'No, I don't need to think about this right now!', make a conscious effort to dismiss it from your mind.

Much of these unwanted thoughts just stray into our minds, not because we want them there, but because we don't do anything to stop them from getting there or staying there.

If we had a filter on the entrance to our minds, it would stop most of these stray and unhelpful ideas from gathering fruit. That's where the practice of monitoring our thoughts comes in, by observing them more regularly, we can decide which ones to follow and which ones we are better to quash and dismiss.

At first, this may seem difficult to understand. Being asked to do something different with our brain, especially once we get past the age of thirty-five, demands a bit of perseverance before it becomes natural to us. Utilising **all** of the exercises in this book is crucial to overcome the effects DMA can have on our minds. Follow this simple guideline:

When you notice any unwanted thoughts of the past or the future in your mind, bring your thoughts back to the present moment and focus on what you are occupied doing in the 'Now'.

Don't beat yourself up if it takes several weeks of practice to master this. Just persevere, you will get there, I promise. As time goes on you will not need to keep pulling yourself away from thoughts of the past or future, they will just naturally stop entering your head as often.

Quashing the tendency to overthink is one of the best ways to short circuit the Inner Abuser's influence because it usually bases its negativity on disturbing things from your past or worries about the future. If we can master the ability to concentrate on what is happening in the present moment, other thoughts would not get the opportunity to enter our heads! As a bonus, if you can distract your mind from the past and the future, you will find you can deal with what is happening in your life right now, much more effectively.

So how do we do that?

Some guidelines to help you stop **OVERTHINKING:**

1. When you are on your own …
… our minds can run riot when it comes to overthinking. Usually, this happens when we are bored or carrying out a mundane task, something we can do without too much thought … like lying awake in bed before we get up in the morning, doing the dishes, cleaning the house or the car, or even just taking the dog for a walk. There are so many times in our life when we don't need to concentrate on the task at hand and that's when the Inner Abuser will take the opportunity to direct our thoughts onto something negative. Something that we don't need to think about, but we do.

There is no guarantee anything we worry about in the future will ever happen, but it doesn't stop us from running over plenty of unhelpful scenarios in our minds, throughout our waking hours. We may find ourselves worrying about what someone else thinks of us, or might say to us, or might say about us … or worrying we may sleep in, miss the bus or train, lose our job or not have enough money in the future. All these ideas and more are present in our subconscious and the Inner Abuser can't wait to use them to start a string of negative thoughts in our minds.

Firstly, remember to check in on your thoughts, and ask yourself these questions,

- 'Do I **want** to think about this right now?'
- 'How is **this** thought making me feel?'
- 'Do I **need** to think about this right now?'
- 'Is **this** thought helping me to make a decision?'
- 'Is **this** thought making me feel good or bad?'
- 'Do I want to continue with **this** thought right now?'
- Finally, 'how good would I feel if I didn't have **this** thought in my mind?'

If you answer these questions and find that your present thoughts are not making you feel good or serving any purpose, tell yourself …
'I am not going to think about "that" any more just now', then practise immersing yourself in the present moment, and whatever you are doing.

When you find you have a little spare time come back and practise this short exercise …

Imagine you are a tiny version of yourself and you are sitting cross-legged, on a stage just above and behind your real head. Now, imagine you are watching a screen on the inside of your forehead. Imagine your present thoughts in print, running across the screen like ticker tape, as they come into your head. Don't try to stop them, just watch them, read them but do not judge them. They are only thoughts, they hold no power over you. Just watch them, as they appear and disappear. What you may find is that they quickly dry up and the screen becomes blank. If that happens just keep watching that blank screen, for as long as you can, and concentrate on it.

When your mind wanders (it will), and you're no longer concentrating on words on that 'screen', refocus on your visualisation and the printed words of the thoughts on the inside of your forehead … concentrate on them once again. Don't judge them, just watch them come and go.

Keep doing this for a few minutes until you get better at watching the screen as it becomes blank and your thoughts naturally disappear from it.

You can do this exercise as often as you like, but of course, only when it is safe to do so.

It's a great way to quieten your mind.

2. When you are in company …
… a great way to stop overthinking when you are in company, is to listen intently to what the other person is saying, hear the words and give the person your full attention. This is not a lesson on how to be more polite, although it generally has that effect, it is a lesson in focusing and grounding your mind and body in the present moment.

- What is this person saying?
- What are they teaching me?
- What can I do or say to help them?
- What are they trying to find out from me?
- What do they want to give me?
- What do they want me to give them? Advice? My attention? My support? My help?

By focusing on the people you are with, you will understand the situation better, and participate more deeply in the present moment.

Give them your attention, but also be aware of all the other things happening around you as well. By immersing yourself in the moment you may find there is a lot more to enjoy in real time.

Even if you are in a difficult predicament, think about what it is teaching you, or try to find any positives, no matter how small, about the situation you are in at that time.

No matter where you find yourself throughout the day, try to ground yourself in the present moment, dismissing any thoughts of the past or the future that might arise. If you have to think about your day, week or year ahead then, of course, you must do it, but once dealt with remind yourself that you do not have to think about it after the task is fulfilled. If necessary, write it down, then your thoughts don't need to keep drifting back to a subject just to remember it.

Finally, for a busy woman, maybe with children to consider, this might not feel that easy at first. Your Inner Abuser may try to convince you, that you *'have to'* think about past, present and future all day long, but you don't. You have been conditioned to believe you have to be thinking every second of every day, just to keep your life in order. That isn't true and the only way you will discover the peace you can create by reducing the habit of overthinking is to practise the ways to stop it, as described above.

If there are lots of tasks to complete, get into the habit of carrying a notepad and writing them down. Once something is committed to paper, the act of writing instils that message in our minds on a more permanent basis. It also stops us from having to busy our heads, trying to remember everything.

All this helps to create a more tranquil mind, but you need to practise it to realise how well our headspace operates once you master this thought-watching exercise.

There are sections of this book you will want to read over again, so remember to underline or highlight things that resonate with you as you go. This whole section on overthinking should be one of them.

Remember, try to avoid thinking never mind overthinking anything to do with your DMA partner. Allowing him into your mind is probably not going to be helpful, so use the above techniques to keep him out.

CHAPTER 7

WHAT FEEDS THE EFFECTS OF DMA AND WHAT STARVES THEM?

If you are serious about overcoming the way DMA has affected you, this chapter should not be overlooked.

You may have wanted to read about an easy way out of a DMA relationship, but the quickest explanation of domestic mental abuse is, abuse of the mind. It's easy to think the problem starts and ends with your partner's words and actions, but it's not that straightforward. They are not the only things that affect the way our brains function throughout the day. If these other things are not addressed, fighting DMA becomes more difficult. If you ignore them, overcoming DMA as rapidly as you would like might not be as easy.

DMA enhances negative emotions, but it is not alone, other aspects of our lives can have a negative influence on our minds too. If we don't tackle them also, our battle to overcome DMA may not be as effective.

When you find the courage to leave your partner and start a new home, you don't want anything to discourage you from staying positive. So, if we are not aware of the influence chemicals in our diet can have on our minds, we might mistakenly believe that a poor mood is due to being alone or away from our abusive partners.

A low mood creates a breeding ground for all the negative emotions that align themselves with DMA. Without being aware of it, guilt and fear can creep in, triggered by substances in the food we eat. Not only that, the constant bad news we are exposed to on TV, radio and in newspapers has a similar negative influence on our subconscious. This chapter outlines the things it's best to stay away from, and also those that have a positive effect on our mindset. Adjusting several aspects of your life will help you overcome DMA a lot easier than following the exercises in this book on their own. This chapter is about adjustments you can make to enhance your life, and diminish the effects of DMA as quickly as possible.

₪

Making some small lifestyle changes is an integral part of the process. The more of these little changes you make, the quicker you can expect to reverse the negative influence your partner has had on your life. If you don't change anything, by default it means you stay the same, making it easier for the Inner Abuser to continue to control important decisions in your life.

Imagine your mind as a set of scales, positive balancing out negative. The negative side is substantially weighed down, to begin with (due to the effects of DMA), and for the moment at least, it far outweighs the positive side of your mind. We need to flip the balance of power to the positive and remove those things that are weighing down the negative side. To do this properly, the recommendations in this chapter should be followed.

Your Inner Abuser might make an appearance about now, suggesting, '… but this doesn't apply to you because … x, y or z'. Whenever this happens, remind yourself that you want to do all you can to reverse the effects of DMA, and try not to let your Inner Abuser decide which parts of this book you will follow, and which ones you will ignore. All the advice in the book is designed to be used collectively, not individually. Bear this in mind if you find yourself less inclined to follow some of the recommendations.

If you skip any advice, the weight on the negative side of those scales in your mind will remain unchanged. Depending on what you feed it, your subconscious will weigh down either side without prejudice, so be careful to ensure all the changes you make are positive ones.

Your DMA partner has had a huge impact, but he is not the only bad influence on your mind.

We all face bad influences every day that feed our 'Inner Abuser'.

To reduce their effect, we have to recognise where they come from and make the necessary adjustments in those areas of our lives.

₪

Anything we see, hear, eat, smell or breathe influences our mind.

Failing to realise this short statement will help keep the negative side of those scales weighed down.

Anything we see and anything we hear.
As we said at the end of the last chapter, you must try to avoid anything you may see, hear or read if your DMA partner tries to contact you. Any communication from him is toxic and designed to weaken your resolve. But what else do you see or hear, that weakens your resolve?

Modern media news is full of negative stories, if you doubt this, watch one full programme of any TV news show. Count the number of stories and how many are 'bad news'.

War, murder, famine, death, poverty, economic uncertainty, mass health scares and questions over public figures' honesty. The list is endless. Almost all of it is bad news.

To minimise your exposure to negativity, you have to limit your exposure to daily news programmes or better still stop watching them altogether. TV, radio, newspaper or magazines; if possible, avoid them all, it will help rebalance those 'scales' quicker.

This will probably take an adjustment to your daily routine, but I promise you, over time, you will not miss it, or miss out on news. Why? Because media news is very difficult to avoid entirely, even when you listen to your favourite calming radio station, the news pops up all too frequently to be able to dodge it completely. I turn down the radio when the news is due to come on, at least, when I remember and can reach the radio in time. Mostly, it's the same news every half hour, and that in itself is a form of repetitive programming. Media news tips those 'mind scales' the wrong way, it affects us in the same way DMA does, by negatively programming our minds, without us being aware of it.

Starving your subconscious of negative stories is part of the recovery process and why a media fast is so good for you, **bad news has a lasting effect on your subconscious without you realising it.**
  The Inner Abuser will attach itself to anything you absorb from the outside world and use it to keep you suppressed, depressed, confused and fearful.
  If you want to recover from the effects of DMA quicker, avoid the media's daily news.

'No News is Good News'. Apart from anything else it simplifies your life and gives you more time to focus on yourself, your recovery and all things positive. Beating DMA is a serious challenge, try not to start being selective with the advice you choose to follow and add a media fast to your daily routine. This advice applies to everyone, not just those overcoming mental abuse.

ANYTHING WE EAT OR DRINK

FOOD AND MOOD

(Be careful with the advice on food and supplements here, and make sure they will not affect any allergies or prescribed medicines you are taking)

To feed ourselves positivity we need to pay attention to our diet … and before I say why you may find your Inner Abuser already trying to undermine this too! Ignore it and get ready for a surprisingly big step toward overcoming DMA …

When we have an ailment or illness we buy drugs from the pharmacy or take those prescribed by a doctor, to help us recover, but very few of us stop to think about what is in these pills and potions, we just expect them to have a beneficial effect on our illness or symptoms.

So what *is* in these pharmaceuticals that are meant to help us? Well in many cases it's a cocktail of chemicals. Chemicals, compounds, trace elements and maybe even vitamins and minerals that we believe are all beneficial to us. Some are meant to help us heal cuts, bruises, infections and physical ailments. Some are meant to help our mood and our mental health but adverse effects from pharmaceuticals are on the increase and it is prudent to explore less aggressive ways to sustain a healthy mind, for our own long-term benefit.

Although the chemicals in medicines are meant to heal us, occasionally some of them have the opposite effect. If we take the wrong medicine it can make our symptoms worse or even create new ones. In this fast, modern world we don't stop to consider that what we put in our mouths could be having a detrimental effect on our health, both physical and mental. To overcome mental abuse we have to consider what we eat and drink as it all has a big impact on the state of our mental health, and our ability to beat DMA. Remember DMA stands for domestic 'mental' abuse.

The pills we take are not the only source of chemicals that find their way into our bodies. We need to consider the food and drink we consume daily too, they can also contain additives that are not beneficial for good mental health. Some of them can affect us physically or mentally and sometimes they can affect both. If you want an example of something that affects both, consider alcohol, too much and we can neither control our legs nor our brain. Too much alcohol affects our physical and mental well-being. It may not be popular, but I highly recommend that you cut alcohol out of your diet completely, within two or three weeks you will notice being more alert, clear-headed and more level-headed too. This is a big step towards overcoming DMA and will remove a lot of weight from the negative side of those scales.

Think of it like this, you don't need to feel you are giving alcohol up for good (although some of you may want to after realising how good you feel without its influence). Abstinence can be temporary until you feel mentally strong enough to deal with any adverse situations. Alcohol is not your friend at a time when you are trying to overcome DMA. It may feel like a crutch, but it weakens your willpower and can defeat many of the positive efforts you made previously. Try not to succumb to 'just one drink' in a moment of weakness.

Alcohol, along with all other legal, and illegal drugs, changes our mentality and lowers our inhibitions, these things will all hamper recovery. Please, try, at least temporarily, to give them up. If you feel this is a step too far, limit alcohol to one or two drinks, on only a couple of nights a week, and have two alcohol-free hours before bedtime. However, this is not what I recommend, but if your resistance is weak, it is an alternative. I will say, though, any use of alcohol can undermine the efforts you make to beat DMA. Bear that in mind.

נ

Other chemicals in our food and drink affect us, even when the symptoms are not as obvious as alcohol. The effects may be more subtle, but they can have a big impact, either instantly or over time. Using alcohol as an example again, the immediate and obvious effects are easy to see but too much can cause liver damage which isn't obvious but still life-threatening in the long run.

Disruption to our state of mind caused by certain food and drink can be subtle, but is detrimental, especially when we are unaware of what is causing anxiety or mood swings. Consider the impact some foods cause when trying to stay positive throughout the day.

When you feel more irritable, anxious or frightened at times, but can't put your finger on the reason, it could be a result of eating or drinking the wrong thing, earlier that day. It could also be, that you are slightly deficient in a vitamin or mineral. The point is, that consuming the wrong food or drink can make it more difficult to overcome DMA.

It's something that is easily overlooked and I'd like you to pay particular attention to this while you work on creating the 'new you'.

DMA creates a negative mindset, and so does eating or drinking certain foods. Realising this makes it obvious that being more careful about what we consume, can help us to overcome the negative effects of DMA.

It is a good idea to be more conscious of the chemicals used **on** our food before it reaches the table, chemicals to create crops that resist pests and diseases, for instance. It also helps to become more aware of preservatives and GMO foods too. Food that has been processed loses some beneficial properties and may even gain some bad ones. Take time to think about what is in the food you eat and the possibility of a detrimental impact on your mindset. The quickest way to beat DMA is to minimise the ability for anything to harm your mind.

This is a big deal.

DMA can trigger food cravings, cause you to overeat or it can kill your appetite completely. Losing yourself in a chocolate-bingeing session will do nothing to help your frame of mind in the long run.

If you notice that your eating habits have changed, then try to understand your thoughts about eating have changed too. Mental abuse can be responsible for both overeating and under-eating. Gorging or starving yourself can be a sign that DMA is manipulating your mind. Controlling what you eat and drink is a good way to improve moods based on your subconscious. Don't underestimate the importance your food choices have on your thought processes. The influence a modern 'processed food' based diet has on your gut doesn't help to promote a positive mind.

Making sure your gut is healthy is extremely important. You may have heard of your 'gut brain', it is linked directly to the brain in your head and both are made from the same tissue during the development of the foetus in the womb! It may be surprising, but the gut brain influences your mental health too. Tweaking your eating habits can help overcome DMA faster, in a way most of us are not aware of.

Remember, we are working on DMA from every angle, we can't overcome something unless we address the whole problem. DMA influences areas of your life you may not be aware of, and one of those is what you eat and drink. That impacts your health, both physically, and more importantly for us, mentally.

HERE IS A LIST OF FOOD AND DRINK THAT YOU SHOULD TRY TO AVOID

Get your pen ready to mark anything here that may trigger your mood.

1. Sugar; Your mood can fluctuate depending on the level of your blood sugar. Sugar **inhibits** a growth hormone in our brain, a hormone that can lessen our tendency toward depression.

Sugar initiates chemical reactions in our body that cause tissue inflammation. In the long term, inflammation diminishes our immune system and our brain.

Sugar (particularly fructose) contributes to insulin resistance which contributes to the state of our mental health too. Sugar, which can normally have a soothing effect, may cause depression in some people.

The secret is to avoid sugary foods that give you an instant pick-me-up, because this will be followed by a sudden slump, an energy crash. And with it, your mood will go down, and you'll find yourself reaching for the biscuit tin again, continuing the vicious cycle.
Start noticing your sugar intake for a more healthy mind.

2. Wheat (gluten); Wheat, rye and barley can harm our mood, increasing the chances of depression and other serious mental health problems. Wheat inhibits our body's ability to produce serotonin (a neurotransmitter) which contributes to mood control, depression as well as aggression. More serotonin is found in the gut than in the brain. This makes looking after your gut an important factor in the ability of DMA to influence your thoughts and your mood. Some research indicates lectin, also found in wheat, creates signs of neurotoxic activity, causing several psychiatric problems as well as depression.

3. Processed foods; There are too many mood-depreciating ingredients in processed food to list here. For a start, they contain sugar and wheat, some in great quantity. There is every chance they also contain artificial colours, sweeteners and preservatives, trans fatty acids, monosodium glutamate (known as MSG), and more synthetic ingredients that can be attributed to levels of irritability and poor mood, leaving you more prone to the effects of DMA.

4. Artificial food ingredients (as mentioned in 'processed foods' above), one, in particular, an artificial sweetener called aspartame is very detrimental to the brain and known to cause depression and panic attacks. Other additives, such as artificial colourings, are also known to impact mood.

5. <u>Genetically modified foods</u>**, GMOs;** There are many studies on the effects of GMO intake by humans. A lot of these studies have linked GMOs to everything from cancers to food allergies, gluten disorders to birth defects. It is an emotive subject, however, we cannot be sure how food will affect us when there have been insufficient long-term tests carried out. To be safe, we should lean towards an organic-based diet as much as possible.

6. Caffeine; (this won't be popular with many but the benefits will be) cut out or cut down caffeine intake, and you may find your sleep improves once you get over the withdrawal symptoms.

Cut out caffeine, from all sources. Avoid coffee, tea, fizzy soft drinks and hot chocolate because of their caffeine content. There's caffeine in energy drinks, those popular vitamin waters and even some chocolate and coffee flavoured drinks. It can add up over a day, and result in sleepless nights when you cannot put your finger on why you're so restless. Switch to decaf coffee and tea and substitute sparkling water for cola, although still water would be even more beneficial. You might feel pretty awful for about four days as you go through withdrawal symptoms (headaches are common), but then you should start sleeping better and feeling brighter. If you can't make the change instantly, try cutting out the caffeine gradually. Strong caffeinated drinks can cause dehydration, make you feel edgy, irritable and cause withdrawal headaches when you go without your habitual fixes throughout the day.

7. Alcohol; although alcohol can briefly produce a pleasant and relaxed state of mind, drink too much, and (you probably know this) you'll feel irritable, moody and anxious the next day. Sometimes a hangover can last two days!

The advice above concerns an entire diet, but individual food choices may make a difference to how you feel mentally and emotionally from day to day too.

1. Zinc; Low levels of zinc have been found in individuals with the worst forms of depression.

2. Selenium; selenium is an important mineral for brain health. It has been found that people given selenium see a rise in their mood, and a decrease in depression and anxiety. Eating Brazil nuts is a great way to get your selenium. Try to get at least the recommended daily allowance of 55 micrograms a day.

Selenium acts as an antioxidant. Research shows that the presence of oxidative stress in the brain is associated with some cases of mild to moderate depression in older people. Whole grains are also an excellent source of selenium and other foods rich in selenium include:

- Beans and legumes
- Lean meat (chicken or turkey with the skin off, pork or beef)
- Low-fat dairy foods
- Nuts and seeds
- Seafood (shellfish, oysters etc. and crab as well as fish, especially sardines)
- Eating fish a few times a week.

3. Vitamin D; vitamin D deficiency is the most common vitamin deficiency in the world today. Around 50 per cent of the world's older population doesn't consume enough vitamin D. It can increase the production of the neurotransmitters like serotonin, associated with mood. Vitamin D supplementation helps to keep a positive mental state. Research found women with high levels of vitamin D had a lower risk of depression. It showed an association between low levels of vitamin D and higher incidences of mood disorders, including PMS, seasonal affective disorder (SAD) and non-specified mood disorders.

Research shows people can help manage their moods by getting at least 1,000 IU of vitamin D a day (although 2,000 is better). Very few foods naturally contain vitamin D. A variety of sources include: short periods of sun exposure, vitamin D supplements and our food.

Vitamin D can be found in:
- Fatty fish like mackerel, tuna and salmon (wild)
- Beef liver
- Cheese
- Egg yolks

The sun's rays allow our bodies to synthesise and regulate vitamin D and a bonus of being in the sun is, that it makes many of us feel good.

4. Magnesium; your body needs magnesium to assist neurotransmitter function that regulates your mood and overall health. Make sure you are getting enough.

Below is a list of foods to Enhance Your Mood

The best place to start to improve your mood is probably not in your medicine cabinet but in your pantry or refrigerator.

The best source of nutrients isn't always supplements – it's food. If you want to feel good, then just eat more from this list … and put them on your shopping list. Your brain can produce its own mood-stabilisers like serotonin – if you give it the right ingredients in the food you consume.

1. Blueberries; many berries contain antioxidants and are great for enhancing our mood because they help make your brain happy. Studies show that the flavonoids in blueberries can improve your mood. **These antioxidants aid your brain in the production of dopamine, a chemical that is critical to coordination, memory function and mood.** Avocado is rich in B vitamins – particularly vitamin B6. And they're such a rich source of folate that 33 per cent of your daily foliate needs are met by eating one avocado and 15 per cent of your daily magnesium requirement.

2. Walnuts; contain omega 3 fats, which studies show, improve your mood. They contain compounds, such as vitamin E, antioxidants and folate.

3. Chocolate; has an amazing effect on our mood, it triggers the action of dopamine, a neurochemical associated with sexual arousal, and releases pleasurable endorphins.

4. Cocoa; contains compounds that produce feelings of elation and exhilaration and has a similar effect to THC found in marijuana. It can also temporarily block feelings of pain and depression. *Eating a small amount of dark chocolate daily can help your overall ability to remain calmer throughout the day.* A couple of small squares of dark chocolate (70 per cent cocoa or more) is all you need.

Do not be tempted to overdo your chocolate intake, though, there is too much of a good thing.

5. Protein in general; a high-quality source of protein – like organic eggs, a piece of Gouda cheese or a handful of almonds – helps to keep your blood sugar levels steady for enhanced energy and mood.

6. Green tea; can help you to relax and unwind. It is linked to lower rates of brain diseases like Alzheimer's and Parkinson's.

7. Oats; are an effective mood booster and they slowly release energy into the bloodstream, which keeps blood sugar and mood stable. Oats also contain the mood-boosting mineral selenium. You can steep porridge oats the night before and add dried fruit and your preferred milk, oat milk or almond milk in the morning, it will keep you going right through until lunch.

8. Bananas; bananas contain dopamine, a natural chemical that boosts your mood. They're also rich in B vitamins, including B6, which helps to soothe your nervous system, and magnesium, which is associated with a positive mood. Anyone with insulin/leptin resistance should check with their nutritionist and make sure they are not taking too much.

9. Coffee; although caffeine can have negative effects, coffee can impact several neurotransmitters related to mood control, so drinking a morning cup could affect your general sense of well-being. Coffee activates your brain's stem cells to convert into new neurons, thereby improving your brain health. If you are going to drink coffee, note how you react to it, don't exceed your beneficial limit, and remember, if you have trouble sleeping, avoid coffee and other caffeinated foods before bedtime.

10. Turmeric (Curcumin); curcumin, the pigment that gives turmeric its yellowish colour is thought to be responsible for many of its medicinal abilities. It may enhance mood and possibly help with depression.

11. Salmon, herring, sardines, tuna all contain omega 3 fats, EPA and DHA, and all play a role in your emotional well-being. Research has shown omega 3 fats work just like antidepressants to prevent depression but without any of the side effects. Take a fish oil supplement from a reliable source if you don't eat fish.

12. Vitamin B; is crucial for fighting depression and will help to add weight to the positive side of those mental mood scales. Look for vitamin B2, B6, B12 and folic acid, necessary for the production of serotonin. Eating dark green vegetables – such as spinach, peas or broccoli – will help keep your levels up. Turkey and chicken contain vitamin B6. Chicken and turkey breast also help increase your intake of the amino acid tryptophan, which the body uses to make serotonin. It also helps to make the hormone melatonin, which regulates sleep.

13. Lentils; are a complex carbohydrate so they aid the brain's production of the feel-good neurotransmitter serotonin. This creates a calmer, happier state of mind with less anxiety. They also help to stabilise your blood sugar levels, keeping your mood even. They're also high in folate – deficiencies in folate have been linked to depression. Lentils can also help boost your iron levels, raising energy levels.

14. Cereal; Calcium has been shown to help reduce your levels of stress and anxiety, and fortified breakfast cereals are a great source, as well as prawns, sardines, tofu and cooked spinach.

15. Fruit and vegetables; Fruits and vegetables contain important nutrients and antioxidants, which directly contribute to your health and health-related quality of life. Eating two or more servings of fruits and vegetables a day is associated with an 11 per cent higher likelihood of good functional health. People who eat more fruits and vegetables feel better about their health.

16. Drink more water; it is important to make an effort to filter your water. Installing a filter tap or even a filter jug will do. There is so much more than just H2O in our tap water, and a lot of it is unhealthy for human beings! Don't take it for granted that living in the Western world means the water from your tap is 'pure'.

This book is designed to reverse the negative impact mental abuse can have on your mindset. If you ignore the impact regularly drinking good quality water can bring, you are allowing one more piece of the jigsaw to fall under the table.

After years of being controlled by someone else, we shouldn't give away control of things that matter most in our lives, and one of them is the control of the quality of the water we drink. Trusting that our water companies are supplying water that does not harm us is one of the things we should not take for granted. Studies have shown a link between countries that chlorinate their water and the early onset of heart disease from narrowing arteries. It has been shown that chlorine can build up on artery walls, in a similar way to cholesterol. Of course, this takes time, decades perhaps, but it is an issue and should not be underestimated just because it takes time to happen.

Fluoride is added to the water of some Western countries and is attributed by some to the calcification of the pineal gland.

The pineal gland is what some Eastern countries refer to as the third eye, it is attributed to enhancing our intuition and 'sixth sense'. This is an extremely important factor when dealing with DMA. We need our intuition to be as sharp as possible, to 'feel' when something just isn't right, and this may help us recognise the more subtle signs of mental abuse. Water is extremely important for our bodies to function properly – and even the smallest degree of dehydration can impair our physical and mental well-being. It can affect our ability to concentrate. One to two litres of water a day is recommended. First thing in the morning have a glass of boiled water and drop a slice of lemon into it.

When making tea or coffee, never reboil the water. As well as reducing the flavour of the tea or coffee, this removes a lot of the oxygen from the water.

You should underline all of the last section, as it's extremely important to drink good quality water. I have a water distiller at home and use it all the time. There is evidence that drinking around three litres of distilled water a day can detoxify our bodies so much, that greying hair can return to its original, natural colour before the ageing process kicked in.

Not drinking enough water can cause mild dehydration and fatigue.

Drinking more good quality water enhances our mental health, and positive mental health destroys the effects of DMA.

When living in Scotland for some time, I was led to believe there was some of the best drinking water available straight from the tap. I can assure you, after my distiller processes four litres and switches off, the residue left in the bottom of it is quite alarming. It is a dark brown/black colour and looks and smells quite awful. I was warned by a learned friend not to inhale the toxic smelling fumes this residue gives off. I always clean it out with a small quantity of citric acid crystals before I use it again. Since I started drinking distilled water, several people have commented on the colour returning to my previously white hair.

A few words on how much to eat and when to eat throughout the day. Large meals take longer to digest and when your body is working hard to break down a big evening meal it is more likely to keep you awake or give you a restless night. On the other hand, having a smaller meal in the evening is likely to give you a better night's sleep. It is equally advisable not to overeat at lunch. The best time to have larger portions is breakfast.

There is an old saying: eat like a king at breakfast, a queen at lunch and a knave at supper. It may not be politically correct in its wording but the message is perfect for a healthy body and mind.

₪

Nightcaps may sound like a good idea to send you off to sleep, but they should be avoided. If you haven't managed to cut out the alcohol yet, try not to have any too close to bedtime, it disrupts the part of your sleeping pattern that you benefit from the most. Even if you get enough sleep, alcohol may still make you feel tired and groggy in the morning. You may not wake in the best of moods either. Feeling positive, awake and aware are all important to you beating DMA, feeling crabby in the morning is not going to help.

One more thing before we leave the section on food and drink. This is not a book about diet, the shape of your body or how healthy your skin is. Nor is it a book on how well your digestive system performs. It's also not a book about improving your circulatory system to avoid heart attacks … so although all the dietary advice above may have great results in these areas of your life, **this advice is solely dedicated to strengthening your mind, and enhancing your ability to remain positive in every situation. That is the only reason changes to your diet are being recommended.** Don't let your Inner Abuser distort these facts. The ONLY reason that changes to your diet are included in this book, is because they WILL have a positive effect on how well you recover completely from DMA.

You will only get the best results from this book if you follow **all** the advice in it. If you don't make changes to your diet, then you may not overcome DMA completely. If you don't beat DMA completely, the mental effect it has had on you can linger with you for the rest of your life. I don't say *will* but *can*. If you find you are resistant to making some changes to what you eat and drink, be sure to check where that decision has come from. The Inner Abuser is very persistent and you have to be vigilant if you want to keep it under control. Changing your diet is a great help to change your mind in a very positive way. Remind yourself, that you can only achieve success with this book if you follow the recommendations in it.

PHYSICAL EXERCISE (no pain involved)

You may say, 'I thought it was the mind we were working to strengthen, not the body?'.

It is the mind we are working on, physical exercise releases 'feel good' hormones and endorphins that promote a feeling of well-being and that is why it is included in this chapter. When we exercise our body releases chemicals that give us a natural high and promote that 'feel good' factor. When we feel good, we feel happy and when we feel happy we cannot feel sad at the same time, it's just not possible for the human mind to do that.

Realising physical exercise can make us feel good, will help you understand why it is one of the changes that are so important to help us overcome the effects of DMA. Dr Andrew Weil wrote a book in the 1990s called, *Eight Weeks to Optimum Health* and the only exercise he recommended in that course, is walking. In his opinion, walking for as little as 45 minutes every day, six days a week, is enough to achieve optimal health.

I am not going to argue with him, that's all the exercise I would ask you to do to help your mind achieve optimal health too. However, if you already do some other form of regular exercise, then keep it up and if you don't, then walking regularly will be enough to do the job. Like everything else, the more effort you put into something, the better result you will get out of it. A quicker walking pace will release more of those 'feel good' factor hormones. So if you start to feel fitter from the benefits of walking, you might want to increase your pace and feel the benefits from even more positive endorphins in your brain.

WHAT YOU SEE AND WHAT YOU HEAR

Nature; This is not a return to the dangers of mass media, but a reminder that we need the presence of nature around us to enhance the new changes we are making in our lives. It may not seem obvious, but if we don't connect with nature regularly, it can also have a detrimental effect on our positivity.

Pets; Having a cat or a dog will help you cope with modern-day stress but it will also help you counteract the stress from a DMA relationship, whether you are still living with your abusive partner or have made the move away from him. If you don't have a cat or dog, it's probably not a good idea to get one until you are settled in to your new home. Pets aren't for everyone, but they can promote positivity, balance and love in your life. Creating enjoyable moments with a pet, walking the dog or having a contented cat around the house will all help to restore harmony in your life.

Sea air; Interacting with nature, whether it is a walk in the park or a stroll in the country, even sitting under a big tree, all help DMA recovery, and another great idea to promote the feeling of well-being in your life is a walk beside the sea. The air near the sea is full of positive ions, and even better, if you walk barefooted you are connecting to the earth, grounding yourself and releasing negativity too. That's not a notion, it's a fact. We are electrically charged beings and a negative charge can build up in our bodies if we do not ground ourselves regularly. Walking barefoot is perfect to do this, but so is just bending down and putting your hand on the ground for a moment. Believe it or not, touching a bush or a tree will have the same result.

Flowers; Having flowers in the house makes most people smile, apart from their beauty, their fragrance can lift almost any mood. You may be able to pick some wildflowers for free when you are out on your walk. There's an added bonus.

Essential oils; Using a diffuser and essential oils is also a great way to lift our mood, all essential oils are concentrated and natural, and when you inhale these oils, they can lift the mood and soothe the mind.

When you get a moment, think about what makes you happy, or what used to make you happy, before the onset of DMA. Write a list and make a point of telling yourself to do at least one of these things every day. It could be as simple as having a nice cup of tea.

This chapter is very important, there are many ways in life to improve our mindset, but as always, we have to make the changes to get the benefits, remember how much you want this new life … how much you want to change.

AND FINALLY … LAUGHTER AND SINGING

You might find this a curious topic to be included in a book about such a serious subject, but it is also an important one.

Laughing helps to raise your mood and experts will tell you that even smiling invokes the release of chemicals in the brain that give us a natural high.

Domestic mental abuse is a very serious issue. Smiling never mind laughing may not be something you feel like doing very often when you are in an abusive relationship. However, hopefully, by now, you have chosen to work towards a solution to your situation, so when you get an opportunity to raise your spirits, allow yourself to make the most of it. Laughter it is said is the best medicine, so for the time being try to choose entertainment that will make you laugh instead of cry, these small choices are far more beneficial to your subconscious and your Authentic Self than you may be able to imagine right now.

Ever tried to sing when you're sad? The words would probably get stuck in your throat.

Laughter and singing just don't fit well when we are facing up to stressful situations but if you can make a conscious effort to reintroduce them into your life it will help you recover from the effects of DMA and that will make the effort worthwhile.

Try forcing yourself to sing when you're sad, it's not easy to begin with, but if you keep it up you might surprise yourself, raise your spirits and eventually sing yourself out of the sadness. Of course, this too will take a bit of effort, but it is yet another way of reversing the long-term effects DMA has.

Imagine if you are tired and have to carry the groceries home, on a cold, dark, rainy night and you find yourself thinking about your abusive situation? It might go something like this …
I have to carry the groceries home (why me?) …
It's raining (why me?) …
It's dark (why me?) …
I'm cold (why me?) …
I'm tired (why me?) …
… I'm being mentally abused by my partner (why me?).

But who says that you need to think about all of these things, even at the moment they are happening?

Having these issues on your mind will do nothing to solve them though, will it? This is why becoming aware of what we are thinking, then asking ourselves how it is making us feel, is so important.

₪

We **can** control what we are thinking about, we just need to practise doing it. We must practise though, we can't expect to get good at anything without practice?

So in the middle of a gloomy evening, or whatever is getting you down, remind yourself that you can choose what you think about.

First ask yourself, 'do I want to think about this just now?' then …

'Do I have to think about this right now?'

'Is this thing I am choosing to think about, making me happy, sad or even frightened?'

Be aware of any influence coming from your Inner Abuser, attempting to convince you that you MUST think about things that are wrong in your life. As you practise it will become easier to recognise when the wrong thoughts are being generated. Once you are aware that your thoughts are the primary cause of your upset, make a conscious effort to change them. What could you be grateful for at that moment in time? If nothing comes to mind then practise singing a song. When we try to remember the words of a song, as we sing, even into ourselves, it focuses our mind, and it can override any negative thoughts in the process. Like learning any new skill, the skill of being happy in adversity takes practice but is worthwhile in the long run. Try not to allow your Inner Abuser to tell you this will never work, it does, but for it to work … you must work with it. Trust this new insight into new possibilities, when you practise choosing what to think about.

It will also help to give you a better night's sleep. Going to bed, thinking about what you are grateful for, instead of what is going wrong in your life is very powerful indeed.

Try to remember, it is *your* mind, and you must stake a claim to the thoughts you WANT to have, or your Inner Abuser will do it for you.

If you can't think of anything uplifting to think about, concentrate on one of your favourite songs, out loud is best, but in this case, singing in your own head is okay too.

Pick some songs you like right now, and write them down, not just the titles, but the words as well. Don't read on until you write the titles of at least five songs you like in this space:

Now, if you have just continued reading, that is not a good sign. Your Inner Abuser just denied you one of the most powerful ways to help overcome the effects of DMA, and it denied you the chance to think about five song titles that will make you feel good.

Our Inner Abuser is always looking for ways to make life more difficult, and when you don't participate in these little exercises that can help your mind, it is usually a sign that the Inner Abuser's influence is present.

Like many of the exercises in this book, it's the simple ones (the Inner Abuser wants you to ignore), that can work the best … so if you still haven't done it yet, go back and think about those song titles, it will make a difference to your subconscious.

Now, when you notice unwanted thoughts in the future, you can tell yourself, 'That is enough for now, I'm going to think about something good, or think about one of my favourite songs'.

Making that continuous effort to 'CHANGE YOUR MIND' will fundamentally change your mindset in the future!

As you work with this book you are beginning to, 'CHANGE YOUR MIND' from the old DMA-affected mind to a new mind backed by your Authentic Self, a new mind that creates a positive mindset and makes change happen.

(If you need any help, then listen to your favourite songs, and if you can, sing along to them. Don't let the world or the DJ on the radio decide what you listen to, play **your own** favourite songs, look them up and keep them with you, on a mini music player or your mobile phone.)

Laughter is the best medicine for your mind, as well as your body … and singing is pretty powerful too.

Make an effort to seek out people, places and things that make you laugh. Comic shows, funny books or funny friends who cheer you up when in your company. Anything that will make you smile is a powerful antidote to the effects of abusive mind manipulation. Your Inner Abuser is incapacitated by the situations that put a smile on your face and disempowered when you actively seek out things that make you smile and laugh.

Tell yourself, 'You have permission to laugh' then go and find something to make you smile, laugh or even sing.

Domestic mental abuse affects the mind, and that's why you may not *feel like* practising any of the suggestions in this chapter right now, but also why you should try to make an even bigger effort with all of them.

If you have been affected by DMA, it is your mind that has been attacked, and the only one in there to change things … is you.

So if you want something to change that will make a difference, it is in your mind that the change must happen. The only one in there is you, but if you decide to follow the recommendations in this book, you will suddenly feel you are not quite as alone in there as you think.

Start implementing all of the things in this chapter today. Why not give them a try, what have you got to lose when you have so much to gain?

CHAPTER 8

GETTING AWAY, STAYING AWAY

Even when you are living with someone daily, you can still be oblivious to the fact you are being mentally abused. After reading Chapter 4 (the checklist of abuse), you may realise you have been mentally abused without knowing it, and it has been a lot more than just 'difficult sometimes'. You can blame your Inner Abuser, while operating under the radar it muddied the waters and convinced you that the relationship was fundamentally okay.

At this point though, many women struggle to comprehend just how devious their partner has been and that leaves them vulnerable and unprepared for the challenges ahead when they finally discover he is a mental abuser. By then, the decision to leave him seems overwhelming.

The worst mistake possible is to warn him of your intentions. If you do, it will change the dynamics of the situation for the worse. He is likely to pile emotional pressure on you to make you stay, not because he loves you but because he has an inborn need to control you for the rest of your life. Incredible as it may still sound to you right now, **that** is the real reason he will do anything in his power to stop you from walking out the door.

Right now, your partner has probably relaxed into the idea that he's already conditioned you enough to make you believe you 'can't live without him'. He may have created a situation where he is in control of all the finances and told you he owns everything and you own nothing. He might have been allowing you freedom of sorts, within the confines of the relationship and his overall control, but if he hears you are contemplating leaving, he will do everything to stop you and as I have said before, there's a distinct possibility the abuse will increase dramatically.

Your Inner Abuser might be telling you, 'He won't do that, he's not as bad as that', or maybe, 'Don't worry, he probably wants out of the relationship too, you can discuss it like adults'. When we are talking about a mentally abusive partner, nothing could be further from the truth. I have witnessed this very scenario …

… On the surface, one woman's husband was acting as if he couldn't care less about her, but when she suggested an amicable divorce, he hit the roof and showed his true colours.

First of all, he said he was going to jump off the nearest bridge, then, when that didn't work and she left him, he called her up, screaming down the phone 'YOU ARE MY WIFE, YOU GET BACK HERE NOW!'

From that moment on he became very menacing and she quickly capitulated, saying she wouldn't be able to live with herself if he carried out any of his empty threats. She had not properly prepared herself mentally for leaving and when he started this threatening abuse, it had the desired effect, she returned 'home' to him.

This was, for the most part, the fault of her Inner Abuser creating 'legitimate' 'reasons and excuses' in her head, telling her why she should return, even though she said previously, that he made her skin crawl.

She gave up on any future happiness based on his hollow threats of suicide and violence.

She had not prepared properly, and her Inner Abuser was still making the big decisions that caused her to capitulate. The decisions it made, created more upset, more sadness, more guilt and more stress, shame and fear in her life.

Another woman told me her husband declared in the middle of a gathering of their friends, 'I know it sounds wrong, but I love my business more than my wife'. (This is a typical tactic of a mental abuser, he was empowering himself, while at the same time he knew it would be deeply upsetting for his wife to hear, especially in front of others.)

In the weeks to come, she decided to leave him, but regrettably made the mistake of telling him her plans. This turned his game on its head. After that he was crying all night long, pleading for another chance, telling her he would kill himself if she left and promising he would change his ways if she stayed.

She left him anyway, and his tune quickly changed again. She had not prepared her mind properly though, and could not deal with this new side of his psychopathic nature. She quickly succumbed to his verbal tirades, threats and abuse. After she returned to stay with him, his abuse escalated to physical violence and sexual attacks. Her life became a nightmare that she didn't have the mental or physical strength to fight.

Examples like this are duplicated all over the world when a woman makes the mistake of warning her abusive partner she is going to leave him.

If you have just realised you are in a mentally abusive relationship, you cannot afford to underestimate his reaction if you tell him you are leaving. I am not saying every woman will suffer the same consequences as the examples above, but if you are going to leave for good, telling him before you go won't simplify matters when dealing with a narcissistic partner. Thinking he will still be reasonable enough to accept your decision to leave is very risky indeed and is simply not worth the risk.

Your Inner Abuser will try to get you to discuss it with him before you walk out the door for the last time, it will call on all the sentiments it can to convince you to talk to him before you leave. Guilt and shame will be high on this list of emotions, it will drag them into your mind, and twist it to see things his way. With the help of this book, you can prepare for this eventuality before you decide to carry it out. The exercises you will find later will make it easier to dismiss the Inner Abuser's suggestions and stick to your previously constructed plan. That plan will be fine-tuned to give you the best chance of a clean break. You will also have the ability to fend off any suggestions from your Inner Abuser that would threaten your future freedom.

Let's put it this way, if you don't tell him, you get to leave without having to deal with any more mental abuse, and it doesn't give him the chance to 'work on you'. But, if you tell him before you leave, you run the risk of him playing on your emotions with promises and lies.

One woman's husband, who had never laid a hand on her previously, locked her in a room with threats of violence until she 'came to her senses'. As mentioned before, the Inner Abuser loves to create drama, fear, guilt, shame and stress in your life. Do you think a conversation with your partner about leaving will bring these emotions into play? If the answer is yes, then why would you consciously cause that to happen? Is it because your Inner Abuser is in control of your thoughts?

Do you think a conversation about you leaving him will bring love, caring, contentment and happiness into your life?

Many women are unaware just how much their minds could already be compromised by an emotionally abusive partner. If this is the case, one of the biggest and most common mistakes a woman can make is leaving her partner without a proper plan.

It may seem a liberating decision to walk out the door amid his latest verbal attack, but it usually never works out. It's probably the worst thing you can do and it's your Inner Abuser that will prompt you to do it. When in a highly emotional state our mind cannot deal with a situation rationally and that allows the Inner Abuser the chance to take control.

It will prompt you to leave in the heat of the moment, without a plan, then later, it will persuade you to return.

After leaving it will start the process of convincing you that you are not equipped to make it on your own and the weaker your mind is at the time, the quicker you will find yourself back under the same roof as the man you were so desperate to leave only a short time before.

In this way, it gets two opportunities to upset you, while it creates self-doubt, guilt and fear as it does so. One woman told me she only got as far as the front gate before realising she had no idea what to do next and returned to face more abuse and ridicule for daring to believe she could leave him in the first place. That same woman went on to leave her abusive husband at least a dozen times, she even managed to buy a house and live there for over a year before eventually, and inexplicably (to the uninformed) returning to the man who had already committed the most awful mental, sexual and physical abuse on her.

This was not her fault. She did not know about the Inner Abuser. She did not understand what was going on in her mind. She believed her thoughts were her own and didn't realise her mind had been compromised. She never realised he had been brainwashing her with the same mental abuse she was trying to escape from. She was not aware that to leave him properly, she first had to reprogramme her mind, by reversing the influences of DMA and strengthening her resolve. Only then would she be properly equipped and capable of leaving without the possibility of ever returning.

Almost all mentally abused women fall into this trap, and that is why it is so important to have a good plan before you leave.

When a woman's mind has been compromised by DMA she will leave her partner at the most untimely moments, unprepared and already likely to be doomed to fail. Her Inner Abuser is usually to blame for this. Statistics show many mentally abused women will leave and return to their partner up to 15 times before eventually staying away, or giving in to remain trapped in the relationship for the rest of their lives.

Watching a woman leave and return to her abusive husband as many as a dozen times or more is difficult to comprehend for outsiders. However, this behaviour is one of the tell-tale signs that she is being emotionally abused by her partner.

Remember, it is something in a woman's mind that convinces her to return after escaping the madness of her relationship. He was not around to physically drag her back to the family home, but her Inner Abuser was around to convince her to return. Can you see how overcoming the Inner Abuser is so important?

First, it will convince a woman to leave, then, it will convince her there is no other option but to return. It sounds crazy but it happens all the time. When she makes the decision to return, it feels like it is the best thing to do, and our Inner Abuser works away in the back of our minds to convince us it is.

It never is ... IT NEVER IS.

This continuous cycle of indecision contributes to the eventual breakdown of resistance to her partner's abuse. Abusive individuals are aware of this (subconsciously sometimes) and use the confusion to destroy what remains of their partner's willpower. Remember abusers are born with the natural ability to manipulate other people's minds in their genes.

It is not until the moment you return home and the door bangs closed that you realise the dreadful mistake you have made by returning. At this point, the Inner Abuser gets a third chance to rub salt in the wounds, creating more reasons and excuses in your head, only this time it will suggest you might have made a mistake by returning!
The Inner Abuser plays a cruel game and one that can repeat and repeat if you don't learn to take control of your thoughts, emotions and feelings.

₪

Strengthening your mind is very important and the exercises in Part 2 will help you do this.

Imagine you already had an incredibly strong mind. Imagine you could decide to do something and never change your mind. Imagine that is you right now.

If you were like that right now, you would have the strength of mind never to consider returning to an abusive partner.

Is that the woman you want to be?

You might not feel like that at the moment, but you **can** become that woman. We all have that strength within us, do not let your Inner Abuser jump in here and tell you otherwise. We all have that strength in us, we just need to do a little work to uncover it. If you have been mentally abused, it's going to feel more of a challenge, but it's still just a challenge, it's not impossible.

Just remember, negative thoughts concerning your abilities are created by your Inner Abuser, and should be ignored. On those occasions always ask if your future self would be happy if you succumbed to the negative ideas your Inner Abuser creates. Your future self will know there is no going back if you want to be in control of your own life and your destiny.

If you are reading this book AFTER leaving an abusive partner, make a resolution right now, not to return and look forward to the exercises in Part 2. As you use them your mind will begin to create positive changes in your life.

נ

I remember one woman saying to me, '… if I saw anyone else in my position, being abused as much as I am, I would tell them to run and never look back. So why can't I do it myself? I don't understand!'

Even though one part of her mind knew she was in a particularly horrific DMA relationship, the dominant part (her Inner Abuser) convinced her that it was impossible just to pack a bag, leave and never return. This woman could not remember all the legitimate reasons she had to leave him, only the excuses why she couldn't leave, that is what DMA does to a woman's mind and her ability to contemplate a situation properly.
In this woman's case, the Inner Abuser's influence was just too powerful at that time. Her mind was so compromised by fear, guilt and doubt that she could only think of the reasons to stay, not the blatantly obvious reasons to stay away.

Reasons to stay rather than reasons to leave are dominant in almost every abused woman's mind. To justify this, her subconscious may convince her to tell her partner she is thinking about splitting up. This will allow him to make promises to change his ways and persuade her to forget about leaving. For a short time, she will feel relieved that this is the case and believe that he means it.

(Remember the easy way is usually not the right way.)

Once a woman tells her partner she is contemplating leaving, his mindset will change. He will watch her like a hawk from that point on, and the chance to make a clean break will be gone. His game and it was always his game … will change.

There is a simple choice, warn him that you plan to leave, and open up Pandora's box, which is likely to create more misery, or decide to go without discussing it and leave when he is not around to save yourself from more abuse.

Whatever your mind causes you to believe at the moment, does not make it true, it just means you believe it to be true. There is a huge difference there. Let that idea flourish for a moment, and then think about this: If you tell him you are leaving, everything he does from that point on will be for his benefit, and nothing will be for yours.

He will not honour your wish to be free, he will only work to secure even more control over you. If he makes promises, they will not last. If he buys you clothes or jewellery, they will be used as a stick to beat you with at a later date. If he promises to change, he will soon return to his old ways. These abusive individuals rarely change, they say they will, but seldom do.

As you continue working with this book, you will start to realise that leaving him without prior warning is (or was) the best decision you ever made.

If you are reading this book and just realising you are being mentally abused, try to stay calm and refrain from running out of the door just yet, any haphazard plan you cobble together to leave, is almost certainly doomed to fail.

When it comes to leaving, organising yourself properly, calmly and logically then going without discussing it, is the best way to succeed. His biggest weapons are his words and his voice. He will try to communicate with you directly, but following the guidelines set out in the next chapter will explain how to avoid this. Of course, your Inner Abuser will try to convince you it's wrong to leave in this manner, but soon you will discover it is the best decision you could make.

A mental abuser will not let his hold on you go easily. The most effective way to safeguard and protect yourself is *never* to communicate with him directly, again. NO EXCEPTIONS. If you can't quite bring yourself to consider this, you are probably not mentally strong enough to leave him just yet. At this time, your Inner Abuser may still be able to make bad decisions while convincing you they are good ones. It's better to recognise this before trying to leave with little chance of it being a permanent departure.

Do not underestimate the power of the mental exercises coming up.

Just remember, you will only get results if you commit to working with them regularly. One jog around the block does not turn you into a marathon runner and the same goes when we are exercising the mind. Practising these exercises once or twice, will not result in the mental strength needed to sustain your determination to create a new life for yourself.

The message in this chapter is this; do not leave without making a plan or without working with the exercises to strengthen your mind beforehand. However, if you have already left by this point, take strength and try to resist any further communication with your ex from now on. The information to come will help you understand this course of action.

Remember the Henry Ford quote, *'If you think you can or you think you can't, you're probably right'*?

If you have finished this short chapter and found yourself saying, 'Yes, but I can't just walk away without saying anything because … x, y or z', then you have put yourself squarely in the, 'I think I can't' camp.

So for now, why don't you cancel that thought, and replace it with something like:

'Although it feels like I can't walk out without discussing it right now, I know there is a way to turn this idea around, and I'm going to work on it as I keep reading'.

If you find this affirmation difficult, try reading it again, ten times … really, ten times. Even if you were unconvinced, read it again, out loud if it helps, until you realise there is a possibility you can find a way to feel good about leaving, without discussing it first. Remember, you have now accepted this man has been mentally abusing you. He has no loyalty to you, only himself. Any guilt you feel about leaving without announcing it is usually a result of your Inner Abuser's influence on your mind.

To consider the idea of leaving without discussing it is only a thought at this point. Why not have this thought that frees you instead of one that traps you?

CHAPTER 9

LEAVING

PART 1: LEAVING MENTALLY

When we say, LEAVING MENTALLY, it means working to create the idea in your mind, that you are no longer with your abusive partner and you no longer need to consider him in any of your decisions. We want to instil in your mind that his welfare is no longer your responsibility.

In your mind, start to believe you are already no longer 'with' him, you have already left him. Create the idea in your mind that he is far behind you, and you are already looking forward to a brighter future.

This is a point where he has no further part to play in your life and anything he says or does is irrelevant, he can no longer influence your future.

How good does that feel?

To do this successfully, it is best to practise **all** the mental exercises throughout this book and repeat them regularly. Not just while you are working to free your mind from the influence of his abuse, but from now on. Making this part of your routine will ensure there is no relapse during any trying times you have to overcome ahead.

This chapter is here to help you understand how important the exercises are, and encourage you to commit to them. It's best to integrate them into your daily life until you feel you can disassociate yourself from your abusive partner forever.

If you have already left him, the exercises will strengthen your mind so much, that you will never again consider going back to your ex.

It's a great achievement when you finally escape your abusive partner in the physical sense, but if you want to live a full and happy life then the effect DMA has had on your mind is something you have to work on too.

Our state of mind is the source of so much suffering. Working to improve our mental resilience is paramount to creating a better life in the future.

Sadhguru, a modern Indian philosopher said,

> *'You have to make it sink deep into you,*
> *that you are the source of your misery,*
> *you are the source of your joy.*
> *Nobody else, nobody else at all,*
> *nothing else at all but you.' (Sadhguru)*

Reading this, many of us will go on the defensive, giving reasons why this statement isn't true. However, if you stop and think about it, factually, it is correct. The misery you feel is not outside of you, it is inside you. The joy that you feel, is not outside of you either, it is in you. Your mind creates it.

Of course, many factors can influence the way we feel, but it is inside your mind where misery or joy is created.

It may help you understand why following all the recommendations in Chapter 7 is so important. External influences have an impact on the way we see the world. If you only subject your mind to the best external influences and keep away from those things that affect you negatively, you will become a happier person.

One of the greatest adverse influences on your mind will be the mental abuse you have endured from your partner. Escaping his influence will remove a huge amount of negativity from your life. Remember those 'mental scales' in Chapter 7? Well your abusive partner's influence is one of the major reasons the negative side is weighed down.

Remember, he is not the focus of this book, you are. His welfare is not the focus of this book, yours is. His future is not the focus of this book, yours is. He is not your responsibility, you are. When you forget about him, you can concentrate on feeling good about yourself. These exercises will help you do this effectively.

₪

It is important to recognise when other people's opinions, are not always helpful, even if they are given with the best intentions …

Before you read this remember the phrase: What other people think of me is none of my business.

When you leave without giving your abusive partner a prior warning, some may say you are not being 'fair'. Their opinion is likely to be a knee-jerk reaction, without knowing all the details of your situation. It is important not to let any ill-informed opinions influence you. One of the greatest prisons we create for ourselves is the fear of what other people think about us. Remember, they have no understanding of everything you have been through and are usually ill-equipped to judge you in the first place. Very few individuals are in a position to judge others in any case, and only you know the extent of your partner's abuse.

So who should you be fair to?

Him, them or yourself? After all, that is the choice.

Who should you respect the most?

You are not responsible for your partner, he is responsible for himself.

He created a situation where you had only one safe choice to make. To avoid any further mental abuse, the best course of action is to leave when he is not at home. His attempts to influence your mind won't stop just because you no longer sleep under the same roof.

When the day comes you must be ready to end all direct contact with him. If you make the mistake of speaking to him on the phone or allowing him any communication after you leave, he will choose his words with one purpose in mind, to convince you to return to him. In the case of mental abuse, his words are his weapon, if you don't listen to them, or read any messages he tries to send, then any further attempts to convince you of anything end right there.

That does not mean that all the abuse you suffered up to that point will not still be in your subconscious thoughts, but it does mean he cannot add any more, while you work with this book to strengthen your resolve.

₪

Sometimes mental abusers will choose another way to play with your mind immediately after you leave. One of these may surprise you;
They may decide to cut all contact with **you**.

This tactic usually doesn't last more than thirty days. It's another mind game, another way to control your thought process, designed to unsettle you.
Make a note of this, it's a common tactic used by mental abusers.

If it happens, try to enjoy the respite it will give you from his influence.

Take advantage of this time. It will allow you to settle into your new home, now that you know what his silence is really about, you can use it to your advantage.

Use the time to focus on this book and strengthen your mind with daily doses of mind-enhancing exercises.
It's important to make a note of this ...

... something in us is triggered when we separate from our partner, and when thirty days or more pass without an ex getting in touch, it can compel us to initiate contact. It's a curious part of the human psyche, but no less real because of that.

Remember this is a possibility and **do not** fall into the trap of contacting the man you have made so much effort to escape.

On the other side, mental abusers that implement 'the thirty-day rule' simply remain silent, sit and wait for their ex to contact them, then spring their trap.

When the woman gets in touch, they pretend to be having a great time, and often this is enough for their unsuspecting partner to ask to rekindle the relationship.

It is unofficially called 'The Thirty Day Rule'. Now that you know about it, you can be wary not to fall for it ... it is only another trick of the mind, and you don't want to return to all his abuse. Do you?

At this time be wary of your Inner Abuser and don't allow it to 'self-sabotage' you.

In the case of abusive individuals, the period of 'no contact' may be longer, but it will not last forever. When he does attempt to contact you, out of the blue, you must be ready for it. You will soon discover how to keep him away from you effectively, after you make the break.

Eventually, these abusers use anything they can to justify a reason to speak to you, and some resort to lies concerning fictitious tragic events. They do not care if you find out later it was a lie, especially if they get you back with them.

I know of one young woman whose partner told her he had cancer. It was not true, he said it to induce sympathy and create concern and compassion for him. It worked until she bumped into his sister some weeks later and discovered it wasn't true. Emotional abusers are capable of the most atrocious lies just to serve their purposes. To be fair, this was not the smartest tall tale, as it was always only a matter of time before this young woman found out the truth. However, it looks like he was not overly concerned about that.

₪

There will be times when you hear that voice in your head saying, 'I really have to contact him, because of … x … y … or z'. But do you, do you really, or can someone else contact him on your behalf, if it really is necessary

As we mentioned before, DMA creates an addiction to intense drama and the need to court danger. This partially explains why a woman will return to her abusive partner time after time. This need to revisit the drama and excitement can be wrongly interpreted in her mind as love for a narcissistic partner. This feeling creates reasons and excuses in her mind to legitimise contacting him. DMA conditions you to accept drama as an integral part of your life. It can also cause you to feel you have lost something when you manage to leave him. If you have been familiar with this type of abuse for a while, your subconscious can actually crave drama, having been conditioned to accept it as part of your life.

When the abuse is no longer around, there is a feeling you have lost something. This can create an urge to recapture the drama, even when the loss was a partner who was mentally abusing you.

It is worth underlining, if you experience some unsettling emotions or feelings after leaving him, don't mistake them for love, when it is merely a period of readjustment. Being prepared for some conflicting feelings at this time will make this transition period easier to endure and overcome.

If you notice an urge to contact him or a desire to find out what he's up to after you leave, remember, these feelings are driven by a subconscious craving for old drama, even if consciously you no longer want it in your life.

When you quit smoking cigarettes, you still have the craving for them, even though you still know they are so bad for your health.

₪

If he uses the 'thirty-day rule' to try to get **you** to contact **him**, your Inner Abuse might create this idea in your mind …
… *'What if something's happened to him?'*

The answer is: If something happened to him, you would hear about it pretty quickly, from some other source.

In reality, the chance of anything 'happening to him' is extremely small, and this is just another sign that your Inner Abuser is still lurking somewhere in the background of your subconscious.

If that thought emerges, ask yourself, 'Why don't I have this feeling of concern for other people in my life, why am I only assuming something has happened to *him*?'

You probably won't wake up worrying about other people's well-being, but there's a good chance you will where he is concerned.

Day and night our Inner Abuser feeds on drama, worry and fear, and when none exists, it tries to create some by inventing reasons for you to get in touch with him.

If you find yourself worrying about your ex-partner's well-being after a period of silence from him, try to rationalise the idea and recognise it could be a red flag. A warning that you are still putting him first, and not yourself. His past abuse can create this default in your mind. Being aware of the game he is playing with this silence, and the doubts it can create in your mind will help stop any bad decisions that could cost you your newfound freedoms.

Remind yourself, that any time you find yourself thinking about his well-being once you have left, means you are considering his feelings more than your own.

॥

Be careful of 'self-sabotage'.

If you confide in others, you may have to listen to their opinion, perhaps based on limited knowledge of mental abuse and your situation. The only important thing is your safety. Not just physical safety but mental safety too. Many people can't help being judgemental, and you may need to accept that some won't agree with the plan you have to regain your freedom, although they may not fully understand the situation.

If anyone is being unhelpful or even negative, it may be best to stay clear of them, at least until you are established in your new home. Deciding to tell *anyone* of your plans before you leave may create unnecessary complications, rather than help you. If you don't tell anyone, no one can jeopardise your escape, so weigh up your situation carefully.

Be careful, your Inner Abuser may see sharing your story as an opportunity to mess up your plans for a clean break. Remember, it loves drama, so you need to be alert. Involving other people, no matter how close they are to you, is a risk, unless you are convinced they will help you, and not judge you.

A word of caution; I know a woman, let's call her Jane, who was chatting with a good friend about their husbands. The friend said she had always thought there was something a bit strange about Jane's husband, at that point Jane let down her guard and began discussing the abuse she was going through and her plans to leave him.

However, this 'good friend' took it upon herself to speak to Jane's husband and whether by mistake or design told him of Jane's plans to leave. The result was calamitous and he escalated his watch over her to an outrageous level. Jane still tried to get away several times, but her efforts were thwarted and her already fragile nature was broken. After suffering threats, aggression and more mental abuse, she was no longer able to put up any fight and resigned herself to staying put. His wrongdoing escalated to physical violence and sexual abuse. Sadly, being so overcome by the situation, she thought no one would believe her story and remained trapped in that relationship.

If you don't tell anyone your plans, no one can ruin them ... except you.

Try to remember, that the Inner Abuser enjoys drama so be mindful before you share your intentions. If you discuss them with friends or family you may not only have to ignore *your* Inner Abuser, you may have to ignore *their* Inner Abuser too.

₪

People may air their opinion, even if they aren't qualified to judge a situation properly, and if you confide in someone else, you may inadvertently expose yourself to unhelpful 'advice'.

Do you want others putting doubt in your head with comments like, 'I think it's best to tell him beforehand', when they don't know how emotional abusers operate? Usually, other people have little idea what goes on behind closed doors in a DMA relationship.

My advice is to tell no one *unless they already understand your situation, are aware of the abuse and are fully supporting you.*

Others may be slightly upset you didn't confide in them beforehand, but good friends and family will soon understand your reasons after you leave. Once you are safely away from him, you might be relieved you didn't confide in friends or family. As mentioned before, you can always drop into Women's Aid for a confidential chat, if you feel you have to discuss your situation with someone face to face.

ESCAPING MENTALLY

Once you realise you are in a DMA relationship it can take some time to come to terms with it.

You only ever get one chance to make a clean break, and you mustn't make him suspicious before this happens. This is why it is important to watch who you tell your plans to and you also have to make sure you don't alert your abusive partner to your plans either.

Remember, this is *mental* abuse and it affects your mind. You need a clear head to make the right *decisions* because they probably won't be the easy decisions.

Your Inner Abuser may convince you to conceal this book in a place your partner is *likely to find it!* ... So be sure to find a safe place to keep it at all times. Yes, that is what you are up against, remember it is working against us to create complications, that's why you have to be aware of your thoughts as often as you can throughout the day.

It is risky to keep this book at home should you suspect your partner of mental abuse. If at all possible, read it in another location and practise the exercises throughout the day, until you can memorise the routine. If he discovers you are reading it he may destroy it, or take it and read it himself, which would be very unhelpful to your cause.

I remember a woman telling me her husband had found her book *Escaping Toxic Guilt*, and after ridiculing her for hours over it, he threw it on the fire. He was aware her guilt worked in his favour and was not going to allow her to escape that confining emotion easily.

Be on your guard.

There are many stories of subconscious 'self-sabotage' when the Inner Abuser is still in control of a woman's mind. Without realising it, some women leave clues to their next move in a place their abusive partner will find them. Some blurt something out in the heat of the moment, or after a drink, that puts him wise to their intentions. On the face of it, it seems bizarre, but DMA works deep in the subconscious and renders us unaware of the danger before we make the most obvious of slip-ups. This is another reason why cutting out alcohol is such a good decision when planning to leave, and in the first few weeks or months after you manage to get away with a clean break. You don't need to abstain for the rest of your life, but drinking alcohol is one of the most dangerous things to do when you are trying to improve your mental strength and plan your escape.

Seeking more information from the charities involved with physical and mental abuse, like Women's Aid in the UK, will reassure you there is help available when you look for it. Arrange a chat with the counsellors there and if you want the best advice, ask if there is someone who is experienced in dealing with cases of *mental* abuse in particular. The conversation will be in strict confidence. You could consult a private therapist, counsellor or even your regular GP or MD for advice too. If you do choose to talk to your family doctor, my advice would be to think long and hard before accepting an offer of antidepressants. You need a clear head to work with the exercises in this book and simply taking a drug that makes you 'feel better' may only mask the predicament you are actually in. Antidepressants treat the effect, not the cause. Using prescription drugs as a remedy to DMA is a very last resort and only for when you feel you just cannot cope with the situation at that point. They can make your partner appear less of a threat to you, and you may find yourself mistakenly thinking you can handle the relationship for the long term.

The other reason I would ask you to be wary of pharmaceuticals is this; if your abusive partner finds you are on antidepressants, he is likely to use this to encourage a sympathetic ear from anyone who will listen. When you leave, he may even say, you have had a breakdown, are not in your right mind and don't realise what you're doing because you are taking pills for depression.

TO RECAP

- You only get one chance to make a 'clean' break from a mentally abusive partner, after that he will be on his guard and will 'invent' as many reasons as he can to convince you that you just cannot leave.
- If he has no reason to suspect that there is a possibility of you leaving, he will not bother planning against the scenario.
- If he realises you are thinking of leaving him, he will try to access your personal data and your private affairs at every level he can, to get the upper hand on you.
- Don't run out the door if you haven't made a proper plan yet.
- Decide to strengthen your mind with this book.
- Without proper preparation, no matter how upset or adamant you get at times, you'll soon feel the urge to return.
- It's still possible to leave a second time (or a third), but usually, it can be more difficult to escape the situation after he is aware of your thoughts and plans.
- If you confide in anyone before you leave you must trust them 100 per cent.
- Unless you have already left, work with the mental exercises coming up, before deciding the date of your departure.

- Once you have been working with the exercises for several weeks, you will feel stronger mentally and more confident to leave and not return, but you must give them time and don't do anything prematurely. It may take a bit longer before you are ready, don't rush it.
- The next chapter has all the advice to prepare and depart physically, once you gain the mental strength to make it permanent.

Finally, if you think you cannot stand to be with him, now that you realise he is mentally abusing you, remind yourself that you have had the strength to deal with him up until now, and survive. It may be a challenge but if you can remain and build the mental strength to plan your departure properly you have a better chance of making it a success.

Domestic mental abuse can create an illusion in your mind that you are in control, that you are not brainwashed, and that you know exactly what you are doing when the exact opposite is true.

By trying to beat DMA on a physical level alone, many women find themselves returning to their partner again and again. It isn't physical abuse they are dealing with, it is mental abuse. Only by working on your mental strength can you put your partner and the memory of his abuse behind you forever.

Only by doing the right things to reverse the effects of mental abuse, and abuse of the mind, will you be tackling the situation correctly.

₪

A word about Women's Aid and similar organisations; by the time a woman approaches these charities for help, she is usually at breaking point. Only a few arrive simply for a bit of advice. Most of the time, they have just walked out on their abusive partner and don't know what to do, or where to go next.

At this point, they are adamant, they never want to see his face again. The staff on duty don't often encounter women who just want to get a bit of breathing space before returning to their abusive partner. Usually, the women want to leave for good. But, if you speak to the workers at these charities, they will tell you that many of the women they see coming through the doors, end up returning to their homes, their abusive partners and more abuse. For some women, this cycle will happen over a dozen times and it is heartbreaking for the staff to see them returning time after time.

To stop becoming another one of these statistics, it is vital to strengthen your mind **before** you leave, and it is vital to **make a plan**.

All of the women who follow the cycle … abused, leave, return, abused, leave, return, abused, leave, return … and every time they leave, they never expect to return, but they do. Their mind has been conditioned, through mental abuse, to act like this.

That's why you have to make a plan and work towards it, or the chance of becoming another one of the statistics above, will be high.

The staff at all of these charities would love to see a day when they have no more women coming through their door for a second or third time, never mind a tenth or eleventh time. Taking back control of your mind is the way to stop this cycle from happening to you.

For a woman, it is safer and more beneficial to talk to someone who is not emotionally involved with the situation, or in particular too close to her abusive partner. If his charm worked to manipulate *her* thoughts, he may have managed to convince some of her friends and family that he is a 'lovely' guy too. I have witnessed an individual convince others that his abused wife was the one with psychological problems.

If you seek help and support from organisations devoted to helping abused women, you can get better, more experienced and impartial advice. Many are available on a 'drop-in' basis day or night.

It's best not to discuss a date of departure with anyone else unless you need their help on that day. D**o not text, call or video chat with anyone about your plans. It is too dangerous to use any electronic equipment to discuss your plans.** The next chapter will explain why.

If you do discuss the date of departure with anyone face to face, make sure your mobile devices, and theirs too, are out of earshot. You will understand why in the next chapter.

LEAVING

PART 2

LEAVING PHYSICALLY
(HOW TO LEAVE YOUR ABUSIVE PARTNER SAFELY)

If you are reading this and saying to yourself, *'Why do I have to leave? Can't I just do something else to change things with my partner?'*, **you may not have taken enough time to consider what has been discussed so far ... but ...**

.......the quick answer is, that *you* have to leave because mental abusers cannot change their own mindset, it is not in their genetic code to adjust their attitude when they are in the wrong regarding their abuse. Many of them are borderline psychopaths or sociopaths, they were born with that mindset and it is an inherent part of who they are.

If you are living with a mental abuser, no matter how bad he is right now, all you can realistically hope for is that he doesn't get any worse, because he can't get better. He can 'act' more reasonably for short periods, but that is it.

Usually, they get worse, and the longer you are with him the more abuse you can expect, over time. Eventually, they get bored just having complete control over your life. In many cases, physical abuse creeps into the relationship and that will also escalate as the years go by. Any belief that your abusive partner is somehow different from the rest will be unfounded, based on hope rather than any truth in the matter.

That may not be easy to take on board, but if you choose to believe your partner could never resort to physical violence, you are likely to do nothing at this time. That belief is probably a result of his mental conditioning. His manipulation of your mind creates the illusion that you are still, somehow in control.

Your Inner Abuser will try to convince you this book is wrong and you know best when it comes to 'your man'.

If you're not quite sure that leaving him is the only way you can find happiness in the future, read on.

Read on, without making any major decisions about whether to stay with him or leave, at this point ...

Escaping mentally, as discussed in Part 1 of Chapter 9, has to be the first thing you work on, using all the techniques and recommendations you find in this book. Preparing your mind mentally should help override any inexplicable urges compelling you to return to your abuser. This is a common occurrence, but as long as you can quell the urge there will be no harm done.

At these moments, the memories of all his abuse are suppressed, and even though, deep down you know he will continue to abuse you, you'll find it hard to resist these sudden urges to return if you haven't prepared for them properly. I watched a woman who told me first hand that she *'didn't even think about him any more'* return to her abusive partner, just a few days later.

The fact is, leaving physically is not the main objective. If you make a sudden and unprepared exit, no matter how certain you are that you will never go back, the odds are, that you probably will. Building up the mental strength you need to make leaving him a success ... is the key. It is strengthening the mind that will ensure long-lasting stability after you leave, not the fact you were able to walk out the door, determined, at least for that moment, never to return.

Assuming you have built up your mental strength sufficiently and feel sure you are ready to leave for the last time, try to put **all** of the following recommendations in place, either before you leave or directly after you leave.

If you find yourself cherry-picking which recommendations you will follow, you may not be ready to make that final move. If you want to make a successful break, it is best to follow **all** of the advice in your preparations.

I remember a woman creating all sorts of reasons and excuses on the day she was packing to leave, while her abusive husband was at work. She had mislaid things and was making mistakes and delays as her friends tried to help get her away from the house, as quickly as possible. Her Inner Abuser caused her to stall, it created a drama by insisting (in her mind), that she found her passport before leaving. The 'Inner Abuser' was still in control, it created this 'legitimate' excuse that she felt compelled to comply with before leaving. She *had to* find her passport.

She knew he watched her all day, via an app on his phone linked to the CCTV cameras he had installed *inside* the house. She was aware he could be on his way home after watching on his smartphone, yet she insisted on finding the passport. Thankfully, she got it and left the property long before he arrived back home.

Even when she was well away from the house, she still managed to give him a chance to find her; by failing to remove the SIM card from her iPad, allowing its location to be identified from another app on his phone. It's very simple to use, and available to anyone with a little smartphone knowledge. It was only after she was asked about the SIM in her iPad, that her daughter managed to remove it before he was able to track it. The SIM on her phone had been changed but not the iPad. It was only by having clear-minded people around her, that the 'escape' was successful.

Her mind was still under the influence of the Inner Abuser. In that case, there had been no time to strengthen her mind beforehand, leaving her vulnerable to his projected influence, even when he wasn't there.

These 'mistakes' were subconscious attempts by her Inner Abuser to thwart the escape. This happens when a woman tries to leave physically before she has detached mentally.

The woman in question continued to use the same email address, and when an inevitable message from him came through, she looked at it and the capitulation began when she read over his pleading messages promising to 'change'.

After the email, she sent him her new phone number and before she realised what she was doing, gave in to the urge to go back 'home' to him. Once behind closed doors, she faced a partner that was determined to make her pay for leaving in the first place. There is no doubt her Authentic Self wanted to leave, but her Inner Abuser was always controlling the situation, making sure she would succumb to the 'urge' to return. Far from helping her situation, this episode broke the last bit of spirit to fight him she had.

When a wild horse is being trained, there comes a certain time when it just stops fighting. The human mind can eventually reach a similar stage as well, where we just stop fighting the mental 'training' that is involved through domestic mental abuse.

Before leaving a DMA relationship, you have to be **fully determined that you are leaving and not going back … ever …** and repeating this idea regularly, over and over again in your mind, will help cement it in your subconscious.

You have to give yourself the best chance of success, the *first time* you decide to leave.

The reason leaving physically sounds like a military operation, is because it has to be like one. If you underestimate an abuser's ability to discover your plans or the extent he will go to make you return to him, you will fail.

The recommendations in this chapter are crucial, if you don't follow them, you may put yourself at risk and fail to make a clean break.

At this stage, it is best to realise you have to put all you can in place to convince him you are not coming back. Many women will try to 'be reasonable' to their abusive partner when they want to leave him. Some will say it's just a trial separation, some will allow him to contact them, from the very day they leave. Trying to 'stay friends' is a recipe for disaster when leaving an emotional abuser, they just see it as weakness and exploit the situation to their advantage. On the day you go, YOU MUST ACCEPT YOU ARE GOING FOR GOOD … and cutting ALL ties.

If you find yourself hesitating over the idea of burning all bridges, it may be a sign you are just not ready to leave … yet. I have watched this scenario play out in front of me, the woman's resistance to severing all ties with her abusive partner was a clear indication to me, that her freedom would not last.

It wasn't long before she went back to her abusive partner, and the scenario that many women encounter after returning soon played out, she experienced even more intensive abuse and control.

I hope you understand now, how important it is to make sure all your preparations are in place before the day you leave, and at the same time make sure you do nothing to make him suspicious of your intentions.

If you have been under the influence of mental abuse for a long time, your Inner Abuser will have been in control much of the time, convincing you with 'reasons and excuses' that you have to stay with him.

For this reason, it's best to assume that it is still going to be a threat to your plans.

On the day you leave, if something pops into your mind that slows you down, no matter how much you feel you need to do it before you go, try to recognise it as a delaying tactic of your Inner Abuser. Leave whatever the issue is, and leave the house … you have a new and better life to begin.

The thoughts and ideas he has planted in your mind over time, are his second-biggest weapon, communication with you, in **any** shape or form, is his first weapon.

COMMUNICATION

The two biggest weapons he uses to manipulate you are his voice and his words

He may use these to threaten you or he may use them to gain your pity, arousing guilt, shame or fear in you to achieve it. **Avoid the sound of his voice and his words, written or spoken, at all cost.** After you leave, if you find yourself having an urge to contact him, then grab this book and use some of the exercises in it to counteract that urge. Do not stop working with them until the craving to contact him has gone and good sense and your Authentic Self are back in control.

If you don't allow his words to reach you (spoken, written or conveyed through others), you are instantly disarming him.

Keep away from him and always think about yourself first. Concentrate your thoughts on your own future. This will become easier as time passes. If you do communicate with him, there's a grave possibility all your hard work to escape will be for nothing.

The words in bold are very important and it's a good idea to underline them with the pen you should have with you while reading this book. When you see anything that resonates with you put some asterisks in the margins. If you don't have a pen or pencil, then go and get one now. It is no use saying to yourself, 'I'll do it later', you must personalise it at the moment you recognise its importance. Anything else that resonates with you should be marked as well. If you are reading this on a device, then use the highlighting facility.

Ask yourself these questions:
- Even if I think it would be okay to tell him I am leaving, is it worth putting myself in this dangerous situation before I go, just to test this theory?
- Do I want to stay 'friends' or in communication with someone who has mentally abused me so much?
- What real benefit is there for me to continue communicating with him on any level?
- Would my future self be happy about me continuing to communicate with him?
- Do I know for sure, that I will be safe if I allow him to contact me after I leave?

Having spent years researching DMA, I know any communication with him is a risk, although your Inner Abuser will tell you otherwise. If you're serious about creating a new life for yourself you cannot communicate directly with your abuser. You cannot continue to live in that 'old life'. You must look forwards from this point, not backwards, you are not going in that direction.

No phone calls, no video calls, no texts, no emails, no letters and no form of social media interaction directly between you. Block them all. Don't forget any you no longer use but haven't shut down. Any form of communication will compromise your ability to keep the focus on your own needs, not his. Ideally, all social media accounts should be closed, and people you wish to continue communicating with should be warned not to share any of your new contact details.

As you read these precautions, your Inner Abuser will try to persuade you that all of them are not necessary, it may ask you. 'why should I give up my social media because of him?'. The answer to that is simple, a mental abuser will use every means at his disposal to undermine your resolve after leaving him. Look at this as a sacrifice worth taking, to rid yourself of his abuse forever. If you are serious about overcoming DMA, deleting social media, at least temporarily, is essential.
Any communication from your ex should be seen as an attempt to further abuse you and should be avoided.

NO DIRECT COMMUNICATION is the first criteria for success. You may well think that is impossible … if you do, you can be sure it is generated by your Inner Abuser.

Not only is it possible to stop all contact it is necessary for your safety and your future happiness. If there are legal requirements for communication, do it through a lawyer or a third party …

NECESSARY COMMUNICATION AFTER YOU LEAVE

Any essential legal communication must be done through a third party of **YOUR CHOICE**, not his. All messages should have a means of recording them, emails or texts can be saved in case they are needed for legal reasons later. It means you have proof of the contact and any relevant information has been delivered to him. Emails; always, always … request a delivery and read receipt with every single one.

Remember though, emails should not be sent via your account, and only through a third party.

He cannot be given the chance to contact you directly, if you imagine his words are toxic to you, it may help.

If he does not reply to your messages sent by your chosen third party, at least you will have evidence he was informed and did not respond. Ideally, using a lawyer is the best, if not the cheapest way to safeguard yourself. Failing that, use a member of your family or a friend you can trust, and will not be influenced by the 'spell' of his spoken words.

His abusive ego will be in full flow, using every tool he has, threat or pity. He may threaten to kill himself or kill you, these are commonly used soon after the initial break and your lawyer or 'go-between' should be made aware of this so that a measured response is returned. Although it may be difficult, it is best to ignore suicide threats, if they do somehow filter their way through to you.

Prepare your go-between for this kind of threat and tell them to remind him of the topic that needs to be discussed and to tell him if he does not stick to the topic, the conversation (written or spoken) will be terminated due to his lack of compliance.

Ideally, ask your third party not to relay anything that doesn't concern the reason for the communication in the first place. i.e. any promises, threats, requests or pleadings, none of that is relevant to your future and should not be related to you. Simply tell your go-between to let him know they cannot deliver any such messages and only the original topic that was agreed for discussion will be relayed back to you. i.e. anything concerning your kids or a divorce settlement.

Many women, who have not worked on strengthening their minds, allow their Inner Abusers to convince them to believe their partner's suicide threat is real. So many times I have been told, 'I went back to him because, if he had committed suicide I couldn't have lived with myself', but I have yet to hear of any mental abuser carrying out this threat.

Do you think it is reasonable for him to expect you to stay in a relationship that you detest, and have a life tormented by mental abuse, just because he threatened you with his suicide? That is a tactic of terrorism and is best ignored. Any response by you, good or bad, will be seen by him as a victory over your initial decision to have zero communication. He said something and it **made you** respond. In an abuser's eyes, it shows your resolve is weak, and it gives them something to work on.

If he really felt like killing himself, he should be relaying this to his own family, friends, doctor or psychologist. This threat is commonplace, and it is best to ignore it and better still forget it.

I advise you to keep any necessary communication to the written word and avoid phone calls, if it has to be a phone call, it must be recorded by your lawyer or 'go-between' every single time. Inform him beforehand that this is the case.

I would also urge your third party not to answer any calls he makes to them, let him leave a message, and even then, only reply by text even if he chooses to leave a message on their voicemail. If he doesn't leave a message there is no reason to call him back. This is a tactic he will use to try to initiate a spoken conversation. Be warned and do not rise to it.

You can take as long as you need to overcome the urge to talk to him and no harm should come of it … BUT … you cannot easily reverse the damage that can be done if you make the mistake of having any direct communication with him.

TEARS, SHOUTING, SWEARING AND THREATS

If he gets the chance, he will cry down the phone for hours if he thinks it will break anyone that isn't resolute enough to deal with it. This is a standard tactic used by emotional abusers and should not be tolerated.

If there is any attempt to deviate from the exact reason for the call, your intermediary should end the call. Once he realises tears won't work, he will move on to shouting, swearing, threats of violence or otherwise, if he believes any of these might work instead. However ANY deviation from the topic of conversation and your 'go-between' must first tell him they will end the call, and then do so if he doesn't return to the subject at hand.

If your chosen mediator has to meet him or visit his home to collect any of your belongings, they should take a third party with them. Before the meeting, they should turn on the voice recorder on their phone, and turn it upside down in a top pocket, where it will pick up any conversation that may be used as evidence should the meeting turn nasty. Evidence of physical violence is easier to prove to the authorities, he will be aware of this, and therefore unlikely to go any further than verbal threats. It is always better to record these meetings whenever possible, either visually or at least by sound recording for your side's safety.

Doing all this shows that you have no intention of returning, not only are you keeping your Inner Abuser at bay, but also you are showing those around you, that you are resolute and have no intention of letting your guard slip or your defences down. If any of your intermediaries indulge him in conversation, they can only tell him what they have witnessed ... 'you appear serious about not returning, and he should forget the chase'.

In your mind, the 'contract' of your relationship should already be torn up and you have no more responsibility towards him.

You must show this determination to everyone around you. You will strengthen your resolve by showing a resolute stance while dismissing any urges to soften your approach to the situation if they appear.

He will be looking for a chink in your armour to exploit, your mission is to make sure there isn't one.

Any feelings towards this approach will only endanger you. Your separation has to be swift for your sake. Abusers like to slow things down to regain control. It is up to you and your side to make sure any interaction needed is completed at the onset of your breakup and doesn't linger on any longer than necessary. Urge your lawyer to push this on as quickly as they can.

₪

So let us return to the original subject, denying communication from your DMA partner after you have left him.

There is every possibility he will try to get other people to do his bidding and ask them to discuss things with you on his behalf. You must stand firm and refuse to discuss anything with anyone you suspect will plead his case. Walk away if necessary to safeguard yourself.

₪

To Recap

You cannot communicate directly with your abuser if you want to escape him for good.

- That means, no phone calls directly to you (block his number, take messages through a third party only and remind them not to entertain anything outside the subject to be discussed).
- That means no texts directly to you.
- That means no emails directly to you.
- That means no one you know mentions his name unless it is to discuss a legal matter.

- That means no Facebook, WhatsApp, Twitter, Instagram or any other form of communication.
- f you get a letter from him, you ask someone else to read it and only repeat anything that needs action legally. This means they don't tell you if he is making threats of any kind, or if he says he can't live without you. If there is anything that they are particularly concerned about, they can pass it on to your lawyer or the authorities.
- **You must understand that removing his ability to communicate with you also removes his ability to further manipulate your mind.**
- If you start thinking you are strong enough to communicate with him, especially in the early months of separation, your Inner Abuser is probably overpowering your Authentic Self at that time.
- It is worth underlining, or highlighting the points above right now. From experience, I know you will have to read them and remind yourself of them many times. Doing this will help you refrain from contacting him in moments of weakness.

THE USE OF TECHNOLOGY

Following the guidelines in this section is pivotal to a successful clean break. It must not be skipped or ignored. Even if you think your partner is not capable of using electronic equipment to his advantage you have to prepare as if he is an IT expert. All your good work and preparation for leaving could be jeopardised if you ignore the possibility he will use technology against you. If he is incapable of using it to his advantage he may employ the help of someone who can.

From your existing mobile phone, note the details of all those people you wish to remain in contact with. If you can, save them on a trusted friend's phone, laptop or pc, or just simply write them down. Be careful, if there is any possibility he could have hacked their phone too, find someone more distant that is willing to do this for you. To prepare in the right way, it's best to imagine he is a technological wizard and proceed with that assumption.

₪

Remember, his greatest weapon used to confuse you is his **words**, either spoken, written or sent electronically. You must also be mindful of him asking others to convey messages on his behalf. This section is designed to stop him from using words against you, do not underestimate the power to undermine you contained in them.

MOBILE PHONE

On the day you leave:
- Take the SIM out of your phone before you leave the house.
- Take the battery out of your phone if it is physically possible to do so.
- Put your mobile phone in a signal-blocking pouch before leaving the house.
- (Purchase this with cash or someone else's account or card long before the day you leave. He may be monitoring your card purchases; it's a common tactic.)
- Do not remove your phone from the pouch until the moment you are disposing of it. This may be at the time you sell it or when you trade it in. Never remove it from the pouch in or near your new accommodation.
- If the phone is in your partner's name then leave it in the home when you depart, or if you forget to do this return it

to him through a third party or your lawyer.
- All this also applies to tablets that have a SIM in them or can be used as a mobile phone.
- On a day before you leave, purchase a new 'pay as you go' SIM card, and a cheap 'dumb' phone, (not another smartphone), that you can just call and text from. It is necessary to return to this old style of communication for a short time. Buy it over the counter and pay cash for it.
- Top it up with cash, to begin with, do not use your credit or debit card to do this, until you have new cards and accounts, to ensure he cannot track your purchases.
- Enter all your main contacts on the new phone.
- Never answer or reply to any number you do not recognise. (If anyone is legitimately trying to contact you they will leave a message on your new voicemail.)
- Enter your abusive partner's known numbers on the new phone then **blacklist and block them all.**
- Any phone owned by members of your family (or friends) that your abusive partner has had access to during your relationship cannot be trusted to contain your number. If you want them to have it tell them to install it with another name beside it (it could be a shop or a business name).

The reason for this is simple, he can track you by the signal from your phone. This is the easiest way for him to find you. If you buy a new smartphone, and he manages to get your number, he can find your location within a few metres, and in some cases even when the phone is switched off. Do not be tempted to use a new smartphone for at least a few months after leaving. By that time, while continuing to use the mental exercises in this book, you should have a good mindset and be ready to reject any attempt he makes to contact you directly.

Tracking you without your consent is illegal in many countries, it is worth finding out the law where you live regarding this. Knowledge is power, don't leave anything to chance or 'think' you know the answer when you really can't be sure.

COMMUNICATION ON A LAPTOP OR OTHER FORMS OF COMPUTER

You must not continue to use the same email addresses you had before leaving. This is mandatory if you want to stay safe. You do not want to be sitting alone in your new accommodation and suddenly receive an email from him. The temptation to read it could be too much for most women who have just made the break from an abusive partner.

You should change all the social media accounts you had before leaving him. If you choose to ignore this advice, it will allow him to contact you, and you may not be strong enough to resist reading and acting on his words. Remember, how close you follow the advice in this book, determines the level of help and change you get from it. If you ignore this advice you could be putting yourself at unnecessary risk.

Close your Amazon, eBay and all other online accounts.

If necessary, open new ones, linked to your new email addresses, and never use similar passwords or user names to any you have used before. I have known abusive men to stand behind unsuspecting partners, engaging them in conversation whilst noting passwords being entered onto a laptop or phone. These individuals can be so plausible, whilst being so devious. **Do not take the chance, open new accounts, or at least use new passwords.**

AFTER you have left. NOT BEFORE:
Inform all of your online contacts not to use your old contact details. It shouldn't be a problem for anyone to wait a day or two to hear from you.

If you are using a lawyer, give them the new 'dumb' mobile phone number as soon as practically possible after you leave, and remind them the number is given in confidence and should not be passed on to anyone without your consent.

REDIRECT YOUR MAIL

Redirect all of your mail, and, if necessary, remember to inform any package delivery companies that you no longer live at that address. You will be changing your online accounts, so those companies should not even have a note of your old address when you set up new accounts.

BANK AND CREDIT CARDS

Make a private appointment with every bank and credit card provider you have. Tell them you believe your bank and card details could have been compromised by the partner you have now left. Ask them to supply you with new accounts and cards. If there are any joint accounts, you can withdraw half of the money in these, but that will have to be done after you leave. (And not by bank transfer, he may be legally able to see all of these account's transactions.) If necessary, transfer it to a trusted friend's account first.

I know of an abusive man who monitored his partner so intensely, that he would call her right after she had purchased anything with a credit card, saying, for example, 'You just bought something from Duncan's department store for £45, what was it?'

It can be common for a narcissist to access their partner's various accounts without her being aware of it. Once he has access to the account he can check all transactions online, on a minute-to-minute basis or set up alerts if anything is purchased with the card. Don't take the chance, change every account you have funds in, and change your credit/debit card details. Failure to do so could cause a lot more problems than the effort taken to switch them.

You will have to inform banks and credit card companies about your change of address, so organise yourself before you make the calls, and ask them to change the details, account and card numbers of every account. If you allow your Inner Abuser to give you reasons and excuses why you don't need to do this, you may limit your ability to make a clean break.

Let me be very clear on this; there is a possibility he has installed secret software on your old smartphone. This software has the capability of recording everything you use it for, phone calls, texts, WhatsApp, Facebook, photos and videos. If you ignore the possibility he has done this, you could sabotage the ability to keep him away from you. Why take that chance? Could your Inner Abuser be courting drama once again?

HE MAY USE OTHER TECHNOLOGY TO TRY TO CONTROL YOU

I know of a mental abuser who installed CCTV *inside* the house so that he could watch his partner all day on his smartphone. Of course, when he installed it he claimed it was to safeguard against burglars, but there is little doubt, that his true intention was to watch her every move. Later, she saw still pictures from the CCTV on his phone. Pictures of her standing naked in the hallway after having a bath. He used the existence of these pictures to taunt and threaten her. Unfortunately, she did not have the mental strength to make a formal complaint, or the police may have been able to seize his phone as evidence of his abuse. They may well have found much more than a few naked pictures.

It's worth remembering this in case there are any recording devices around when you are being emotionally (or physically) abused. Many people have a dash cam, and some may have an audio recording facility on them too. Abusers are using technology more and more these days.

It's worth considering if you can use it to protect yourself against your abuser too. If the police act swiftly and obtain his laptop, mobile phone, CCTV, dash cam or other recording devices, they may find enough evidence to prove abuse both mental and physical, and then act quickly. I am not saying this is needed in every case of mental abuse, but it is a reality in some, so don't discount it easily.

It can be a big struggle with your Inner Abuser to justify reporting an abusive partner to the authorities. It's worth remembering you are protecting him while ignoring your own safety if you continue to cover up his wrongdoing. If there is evidence recorded on any piece of equipment, it is the best evidence to keep him from harassing you from that day on. Although it is difficult to find the courage to report his abuse, ignoring the chance to do so just allows it to continue. And why would you want the abuse to continue? What could be stopping you from reporting any of his abuse?

You don't need to do any more than consider this last paragraph for a little while, even if it only makes you aware this is a real option for you, and no more.

Your Inner Abuser will give you as many reasons and excuses as it needs to stop you from reporting him. If you heed these excuses, they will all work in your ex-partner's favour, not yours. Be aware of any ideas in your mind, that safeguard him and not you.

Any feelings of guilt concerning this situation are generated by the Inner Abuser. It will try to stop you from putting an end to the abuse because it thrives on your distress. This is when you'll know how well the exercises in this book are helping. If you can't quite bring yourself to report his abuse to the authorities, keep practising the mental exercises, until you can. The day will come when you realise that reporting him is the very best way to rid yourself of his attention forever. It may not be today and that's okay, but that day will come if you continue to work with the exercises in this book.

If you are reading this for the first time then any resistance to reporting him is understandable. Don't lose heart, the mental strength and benefits from the exercises take time to kick in, and no one can expect to change overnight. It's not realistic for you or anyone else to expect instant results. These exercises are no different from exercises you would use to develop your body, except that they are developing your mind. Any change takes time, so don't give up on them … they work every time, as long as you keep regularly repeating them, they will work.

It can take abusive individuals years to influence the way you see the world, so an expectation of instant results is unrealistic. The good thing is, that using these exercises daily may only take weeks, not years, to start having a positive effect on your mindset.

It's now time to consider using any technology available to safeguard yourself.

YOU CAN USE TECHNOLOGY TO YOUR ADVANTAGE TOO
One Woman's Story

This woman had been married to a mental abuser for nearly 40 years. Even after they split up and the divorce was over, he was still following her with a tracker she discovered on her car. Like most DMA abusers, he was obsessed with controlling her and wouldn't stop harassing her, continually making excuses to turn up at her door, day or night.

During the latter years of their marriage, he added physical and sexual abuse to his repertoire.

One night, he arrived at her new house well after midnight, and after a heavy drinking session. They had a long conversation through the closed front door, but eventually, he talked her into opening it.

Once inside, he grabbed her, and although she tried to fight him off, he overcame her. He then proceeded to physically and sexually assault her. Afterwards, she finally managed to persuade him to leave. However, that was the last time he would get close to her after nearly 40 years of abuse …

Before she opened the door to him she operated the voice recorder on her smartphone. It captured the conversation, her protestation and the noises of the assault. She called the police, and after gathering more evidence from witnesses to previous assaults on her, a short court case ensued where he was sentenced to jail for five years. There was also a restraining order put on him. He was not allowed to come within 500 metres of her once he was released from jail.

This woman would never have married him if she had any idea how the future of that relationship would turn out. But it took nearly *forty* years to finally rid herself of him and his abuse. That is the extent DMA can affect a woman's mind and her judgement over a long period of time.

Finally, by using her phone to record the attack, she felt she had enough evidence for the police to take her seriously. Even though they are more active in dealing with mental abuse these days, this woman's Inner Abuser had convinced her, that they would not be interested until that night she finally recorded evidence for them.

If you do decide to press charges on your abusive partner, the more evidence you have, the better. If you can safely use modern technology to gather proof of his abuse, it is good evidence for the police and they can consider the situation more clearly, from the start. Text messages, and video or audio evidence tell their own stories. Screenshot any text evidence and send it to a trusted friend or family member so that you have copies of it all. You can download free apps that will record your phone calls as audio files, these too can be sent to a trusted third party to be used as evidence later.

If you do not make copies of the evidence then lose your phone, the evidence is gone and your story could be less credible. Make sure you back it up, but not to a 'cloud' account he might already have access to, without your knowledge.

NEW ACCOMMODATION

Once you have decided to leave, start considering where you are going to live next.
The best decision, the safest decision, and the one that will show real intent to all those around you is to move as far away from him as possible.

When you read this at first, the natural reaction is to think of the difficulties involved in such a decision. That's one of the reasons it's best to give yourself as much time as practically possible to consider where you are going to live.

Your Inner Abuser will employ reasons why moving far away isn't that easy. Try not to let this dissuade you, you are only **considering** all possibilities at the moment. You are not committing to any of them at this stage. Have an open mind and think about **all** of the possibilities you have, but may not have considered yet.

Do you have any trusted friends or relatives in other towns, that you might be able to stay with? Even in the short term. If you can't stay with them, could they help you find a place to stay, near them? I know one woman who took an overseas holiday for a month, it meant she was so far away he simply couldn't get to her, at least physically. Of course, there is no point in doing this if you are not strong enough to resist contacting him while you are away. This is why it is important to visualise a life away from him *before* you leave. There is no point in going through all the drama of leaving if you are not mentally strong enough to stay away forever.

Imagine life, without him in it.

Remember Henry Ford; 'If you think you can, or you think you can't, you're probably right.'

In your mind, you must think **you can** walk away from him forever before you leave. Of course, it may come with a hint of fear attached, but as your mind grows stronger, you can put that to one side and replace it with a newfound enthusiasm for a better future without him.

Use all the exercises in the book to fortify your determination, to leave, and leave for good.

Sadly, the woman who took the extended holiday had not prepared to leave properly, she opened an email from her abuser on the second day she was away, replied and promised to phone him every day (from her new phone) until she returned home at the end of the month.

She had two friends away with her but didn't tell them she was in contact with him, so they were unable to help the situation. They believed, that after what she went through to get away, she would never go back. Unfortunately, they didn't know how much the DMA had damaged her mind. This woman had organised an apartment to live in when she returned home. Her twenty-two-year-old daughter, who despised her stepdad, was already living there and waiting for her mum to come 'home'. While she was away, this woman continued to tell her daughter she was coming 'home' to the apartment. But when her plane touched down, she was picked up by her abusive husband and went back to their house with him. Her daughter waited up all night, believing something had happened to her mum before receiving a text from her in the morning saying she was back with her abuser.

Many stories reinforce the need to strengthen your mind and put everything in place beforehand, mental and physical, to ensure when you leave, you leave for good.

It is easy to make the same mistakes as this woman, follow all the recommendations properly, and make sure **your** departure succeeds, where hers failed.

₪

One of the best ways to safeguard yourself, and your kids, if you have any, is to put distance between you and your abusive partner. This, above all, makes it difficult for him to 'pop by', or turn up out of the blue (if he discovers your new address). A common mistake is to take accommodation too close to where your abusive ex lives.

If this is the first time you have thought about putting distance between you and him, it's worth considering the benefits as you read on.

A woman told me about her daughter who moved 400 miles away to be with her new partner. This woman was very vigilant and had already spotted some signs of DMA in her daughter's relationship. So much so, that she made the 800-mile round trip by train every other weekend to monitor the situation. When the mental abuse increased, she eventually managed to talk her daughter into returning home.

This woman told me that the distance was one of the biggest reasons her daughter did not return to her abusive partner. Not only did the distance keep him away from stalking her, but it also quelled her Inner Abuser's influence on her to return to him.

Putting distance between you and your abuser is always beneficial. If he found out where you lived, it would be a long trip for him to try to see you in person. It would also be difficult for him to justify being in your area for anything else, should you need to inform the police that he was harassing or stalking you.

It doesn't need to be 400 miles, even twenty miles gives him a forty-mile round trip, and it's amazing how much of a deterrent this can be. Of course, the further the better.

If you can't bring yourself to move far away, it is worth moving to the other side of town, if he does find you, he will have to visit an area he might be unfamiliar with. Sometimes these individuals can be put off by just that. They may act macho when mentally abusing their partner, but being out of their 'comfort zone' can unnerve them too. If you can strike up a friendship with your new neighbours, they are more likely to assist you, if you needed any help.

However convenient it may seem, moving to accommodation close to him is a big mistake. It makes it far too easy for his unwelcome presence to arrive at your door.

Everyone gets a bit bolder if they've had a few drinks, and if you are within a short taxi ride of his local pub, his mind, distorted by alcohol, could contemplate turning up at your door, late at night.

If he discovers your new address, moving far away means a long trip if he wants to see you face to face.

₪

Whether you decide to rent a place or stay with a friend, it's best to make arrangements well in advance. **Do not** use any of your existing electronic devices to do this. If you use them to search for rental apartments or call agencies to discuss contracts, your plans could be discovered even before you try to leave. Search history can be found on some devices even if you delete it. Phone calls can be recorded or listened to live, without your knowledge.

If you have to look for rental accommodation, do it at an internet café or on the phone, tablet or PC of a trusted friend. If you have to give rental agencies any contact details, ask your friend to say you are staying with them, and all mail or calls, texts or messages should be sent to them, not to your present home address.

Do not give them your 'home' address for any reason. If they don't have it ... they can't use it if they make an admin mistake.

On no account should your friend discuss anything with you on the phone, unless you have already bought a new 'dumb' mobile phone (purchased by cash and topped up by cash too). Of course, this should only be turned on when safe to do so. Don't ever use it in the house you are planning to leave. Tell your confidant, well in advance, you will only reply or contact them when it is safe to do so. It has to be this way. Can you imagine what would happen if this phone rang when *he* was with you?

If they want to discuss your situation and your preparations to leave, your confidant should not contact you on any device your partner has had access to in the past. **Even if he is not around, never use your existing smartphone to discuss your plans in calls, texts, emails or any other form of messaging.**

As unlikely as it may seem to you, there is every possibility your abusive partner could have installed an app on your phone that can record everything you use it for; phone calls, texts, WhatsApp, Facebook, Instagram, photos and videos.

Try to avoid keeping your new 'dumb' phone in your house or your car. It's better to assume he will find it.

Your Inner Abuser will attempt to make you believe …
- 'He's not that smart'.
- 'He won't be checking my electronic stuff'.
- 'He doesn't have access to my private emails'.
- 'He doesn't even know how to work a smartphone properly'.
- 'He'll be glad when I leave, so I don't care if he finds out'.

I have seen all of these things sabotage women in the past. If he gets wind of your plans, the cat is out of the bag and he will probably double his watch over you. If he discovered you were planning to leave he is likely to use it against you, time and time again … 'Remember you were planning to leave, without even telling me! I need to watch you!'. They use repetition like this, to instil guilt, doubt and fear in you.

If you have to give a property rental agency your previous address, make sure they understand your circumstances, and that you do not want any correspondence sent to that address, or you could tell them you split up acrimoniously and you do not want to give out these details for safety reasons.

You can also discuss putting the rental in a friend's name and address if it is possible. It must be stressed though, that everyone around, even your friend's children, know they cannot reveal your whereabouts to anyone else, rumours can spread like wildfire.

I have heard stories of abusers saying they need to get in touch because of an emergency or a terrible accident (it was always a lie, no matter how elaborate the story of the 'accident' was). Those you have trusted, have to know not to give your 'ex' any of your contact details.

There are too many personal scenarios to cover in this book, the main point is not to give out your **previous** address, emails or contact numbers to anyone you have to deal with once you have left him. If they do not have it, they cannot make the mistake of sending any of your private information to it by mistake!

FRIENDS AND FAMILY

Be very selective about who you give your new contact details, and this includes those closest to you. Parents and older people can innocently write your details, appointments or arrangements on their calendars, in their diaries or even on pieces of paper they leave by the phone in their own homes.

I remember one woman's abusive partner 'innocently' visited her elderly mother, once inside the house he took photos of the calendar hanging on the wall. He was waiting outside the mother's house on the next date his estranged wife had arranged to visit her mum. Sadly, once they were all in the house, her mother, who didn't realise the extent of the abuse, took his side and said to her daughter she should try to save the marriage. The abused woman ended up capitulating to this extra pressure and was soon back at the marital home, where, she said, he repeatedly raped her in the days and months to come. Up until then, his abuse had not been physical, the fact she had tried to leave him was enough to escalate the situation to sexual and physical abuse. In his mind, he was teaching her a lesson, and being her husband was fully justified to do so.

It's worth considering, that when you distribute your new details to *anyone*, you make yourself more vulnerable.

The more people you share your new address, phone number, email or social media identity with, the more chance there is that someone, even if it is innocently, will pass on your details to your abusive ex.

There is a setting, even on cheap mobile phones, where you can call those you love and withhold your number. This gives you a chance to explain why you want to keep your contact information to yourself for the first few weeks or months. If people don't have your details, they simply can't be forced or tricked into passing them on.

Mental abusers will lie about accidents or illness in a bid to obtain your details from unsuspecting friends and relatives, if you don't give them your details for the first few months, they cannot give them to him. In this way, you give yourself some breathing space in the initial period after leaving.

If you have children, even grown-up ones, be careful, even they can be taken in by a mental abuser's charms, threats or tears, whether he is their biological father or not.

The need to keep your new contact details safe applies to your place of work too. Only share what you need to with them, and try not to reveal any new contact details unless necessary. Prevention is better than cure.

SEEKING LEGAL ADVICE

If you want to make your initial separation legal in the eyes of the law, then it is best to use a lawyer. I would recommend you find one that has experience in dealing with abusive relationships. They understand the way DMA can affect a woman's decisions better than others and are aware of the coercion tactics these abusive individuals use.

If you share accommodation or other assets with your abuser you may need to seek legal advice to ensure you get what you are legally entitled to in a separation.

One of the advantages of cutting all communication with your DMA partner is that he cannot threaten you concerning the legal division of assets. I know one woman who did not claim her share of the family home, because her abusive partner threatened to kill her if she did. He was already physically abusing her by the time she left, and his threat was convincing enough, to make her feel she could not take the chance.

If you do need a solicitor, the volunteers at your nearest Women's Aid or a similar charity for abused women may be able to recommend one that specialises in DMA situations.

Ask your lawyer what items you are legally allowed to take with you, on the day you leave. Be careful you don't blurt out any legal advice you're lawyer has given you if you have an argument with your partner in the days leading up to your departure. Anything you say could alert him to your intentions.

Any legal advice you receive is best not shared with anyone, at least in the short term.

I know of one situation where an abused woman told her 'friends' that she would be financially well off after the divorce because her husband's business was part of the marital assets. Not only did one of the 'friends' report this back to him, this 'friend' then began to undermine the woman by telling her (and others) she didn't deserve half of his business assets!

These two women had known each other for thirty years, however jealousy in friendships is common, and it can make people do strange things. Be warned about confiding in others, until everything is secured to your benefit and satisfaction.

It may be worth asking your lawyer to construct a letter to leave for your partner on the day of departure. In it, you can request he only contacts you for legal reasons and does this through your lawyer (or third party of your choice). You may also want to intimate that you will inform the authorities if he tries to contact or confront you in person. Depending on just how severe your situation is, you may want to consider serving him with a court injunction that threatens criminal charges or legal proceedings should he break the terms of the document.

It is worth remembering, many lawyers, clever as they are, do not completely understand the extent DMA affects a woman's mind. Because of that, they may question your choice of action, or why you need to leave without informing your partner of your intentions. Regardless of their thoughts, it is always safer to leave without telling him you are going. DMA affects a woman's mind more than most people understand, and even lawyers can underestimate these situations, regardless of their best intentions.

ON THE DAY YOU LEAVE

You must decide to leave at a time you know for sure, your DMA partner is not going to be around. This is very important. Mental abusers can become physically violent when they are triggered and it is simply not worth taking the chance. They can also be very persuasive, making elaborate speeches about how they'll change and never abuse you again. They will say anything if they think you'll change your mind, but it's likely they won't mean one single word of it. They can be very persuasive, and believable when they need to be. That's another reason why you cannot afford to inform him of your intentions. Your Inner Abuser will keep trying to convince you to discuss it with him, but there is no benefit to you whatsoever in doing this. On your departure, you can leave him a note (from you or your lawyer), but make it short and to the point. Take a picture of the wording, and the note lying in a conspicuous place where he cannot say he didn't find it.

This is more important than you realise, it is a distinct possibility he will try to contact you right away. If you follow the recommendations here, it will be impossible for him to call, message or email you, because you will have changed your contact details, numbers and email addresses. Or, you will have blocked *his* numbers and email addresses. The latter should not be seen as a solution, more of a quick fix on the day you leave.

When he cannot reach you, he may pretend he never found the note and try to contact your family or friends, saying you haven't come home and he is worried. If this happens you can share the picture of the note and where you left it. If nothing else this will serve to show others, he is capable of manipulating their minds too, using deception and fabrication of the truth. I am not saying this will happen, but if it does, you have the evidence to prove the truth of the matter.

It isn't easy to accept, but sometimes others have to see the proof before they are convinced by your story. The more proof you have of his willingness and ability to manipulate their impression of the truth, the easier it is to convince them of his powers of deception. It may also help them to understand how he could manipulate you, within the relationship, while pretending to be someone he is not, to gain your trust and your love.

It takes a lot of research and study to understand the effects of mental abuse properly, sometimes even legal professionals find it difficult to fully comprehend what DMA can do to a woman's mind ...

I recall a situation where a woman decided that the only way she could relax after leaving was to leave the country (yes, really). Her solicitor, who did not understand the full psychological effects of DMA, couldn't understand why she thought this was necessary.

A couple of days after leaving, the abusive partner called her. Since the woman didn't know the protocol in this book, she answered and spoke to him, to try to explain why she had left. He called her back later that day and said he had traced her mobile phone signal and was flying out to 'come and get her'. She could hear an airport's Tannoy system in the background, announcing flight times*. Understandably, she was terrified ...

From then on, she believed he was lurking around every corner. By the time she flew home, her nerves were shattered and she went back to live with him, fearful of what he would do if he caught up with her. The lawyer, knowing the details of her case, could not understand why she had gone back to him. Even some professionals, who don't understand the impact DMA can have on the mind, are ill-equipped to represent you properly. This is why using a lawyer that works with local women's charities can be very beneficial. If you are going to use one, choose them well, a lawyer friend of a friend may be well-meaning, but unable to assist you with the unique challenges involved in your case.

*Incidentally, the noise of the airport Tannoy system was coming from his laptop when he made the call, he wasn't in the airport, let alone waiting on a flight to come and get her.

INFORMING THE AUTHORITIES … AT LEAST JUST CONSIDER THIS
(you don't have to do it, just read about it)

If his abuse is bad enough for you to leave him, it may be time to consider informing the police of any concerns you may have about him approaching you after you depart.

If you have feelings of fear or anxiety regarding him contacting you or turning up at your new accommodation, it may be time to think about asking the police to talk to him and deter him from approaching you. Usually, at this stage, they will only make a report that he has been spoken to. If he ignores their warning and tries to contact you, it will escalate the incident and they may refer him to the courts to consider the situation. The court may then serve him with a restraining order.

If he chooses to contact you after the police speak to him, he has also chosen to deal with the resulting actions of the police. You are not to blame for the course of action he chooses to take in life, he is. HE will be solely responsible for any actions the police or the courts take from that moment on. Settle these facts in your mind, you are only acting to preserve your own physical and mental health and safety. Taking back the responsibility for your own well-being.

If he didn't do anything wrong, he would have nothing to worry about. **You are not responsible for him.**

Your Inner Abuser will try to convince you that …
- He's not been bad enough to report it to the police *(if you are scared, then he has been)*.
- He hasn't hit you, so it's not a crime *(in many countries DMA is a crime)*.

- The police won't believe you *(the police <u>will</u> take you seriously and speak to him)*.
- The police don't have time for this *(the police are now treating mental abuse as seriously as physical abuse in many countries)*.
- He has not always been abusive *(it is only now that matters)*.
- He isn't always abusive *(this constant change of mood is actually <u>part</u> of the mental abuse)*.
- He did do some nice things for you in the past *(to confuse you in the present time)*.
- He doesn't deserve to go to prison *(it's not likely to happen, however, the severity of his abuse may decide this)*.
- He might get better in the future *(this is very unusual and unlikely)*.
- He might just leave you alone soon *(classic abusers can continue intermittent mental abuse for years unless they are spoken to by the authorities)*.

Your Inner Abuser will use more reasons and excuses to deter you from informing the police because it wants the fear and anxiety to continue (it feeds off it). Unfortunately, one effect of domestic mental abuse causes the mind to resist reporting a partner.

- Imagine a computer virus called DMA that sabotages the system and installs a safety device, to protect itself from the inside.
- Imagine it was possible to install that DMA virus in the human mind.
- Now imagine it is the human mind that is sabotaged, but the virus installs a safety device to protect itself from deep inside your mind.

- That's how domestic mental abuse works. Protecting the abuser from inside the woman's mind.

This is why a woman finds it difficult to do or say anything that could harm the man that has been mentally abusing her. It has little to do with her true emotions, and everything to do with the way his mental abuse has sabotaged her thought process.

₪

Deciding to inform the authorities about his abuse is one of the biggest challenges a woman faces when leaving the relationship. It is perplexing for the outsider to observe because reporting the situation to the police could prevent any further abuse from then on.

One way to get over this is to ask yourself the question, 'Who do I respect the most, my abuser, or myself?'

If you respect him more, you will look after his well-being. If you respect yourself more, you will look after your own. Doing something to safeguard yourself from further abuse, is not doing something to threaten his well-being. It is merely looking after yourself.

Picture it this way for a moment …

From the time the police ask him to stay away from you, he is in control of his own actions, if he chooses to gamble with the situation, then it is his choice, not yours.

The police can ask him not to contact or confront you, if he ignores their warning, it may become a criminal matter. If that happens, he is completely to blame, not you. If he ignores their request to keep away from you, any future call you make to the police will be treated as a priority.

If you don't inform the police of the situation, and he does approach you in the future, they will have to ascertain who is to blame for any incident at that time. You have a lot to gain, and equally a lot to lose. Take the opportunity to explain your situation to the police shortly after you leave.

Many countries now recognise mental and emotional abuse as a crime, it's worth a phone call to ask the authorities in your country if that is the case. Try not to let your Inner Abuser assume you already know the answer to this question. If you don't want to phone the authorities then call Women's Aid or a similar organisation and ask them.

If you know he is committing a crime, you may feel differently about reporting DMA.

That one call can guide you. Realising that what he has been doing to you is not just 'part of a difficult relationship', but is a crime, may help you see the situation in a whole new light.

THIS DOES NOT MEAN ASKING THE POLICE TO THROW YOUR PARTNER IN JAIL

It only means asking the authorities to make a note of your circumstances and concerns about your safety based on his previous threats. When you call them, ask for an incident number so that you can refer back to the call if you have cause to contact them again in the future. When you call make a note of the name of the person you speak to, the time and the date and of course the incident number. If you can, ask someone else to keep a note of these things too. Women who have been mentally abused can be forgetful at times and it's nice to know someone else has a note of important details for you too.

You are also safeguarding yourself by reporting the situation first, if you don't, your partner may report you. That is no joke, but a real possibility with a lot more repercussions than you might think at first.

*In one instance I recall the abuser reporting the situation first, telling the police that **they** were the one being abused and intimating a concern over their partner's mental health too. The abused person then became the accused, and with that came suspicion and doubt on the part of the authorities. It made life ten times worse, simply because they were the first to be accused of abuse, to the authorities.*

Underestimating the devious mind of a mentally abusive partner can cause more upset than you may first realise.

If you still don't feel up to reporting the situation at this time, it might be a good idea to read this section again, it could save you a lot of heartache in the future.

Since the police are only human, they can find it difficult to discount the first report of events, and it may make it difficult for you if you have no concrete proof your partner has been lying to them.

I strongly advise you to contact the authorities on the day you depart, it may turn out to be the safest advice you find in this book.

- Tell them you have concerns over your future safety, stating you have been living with your partner or husband who has been emotionally abusing you for a long time.
- Tell them you do not want him arrested or charged for the time being.
- But ... ask them to note the details and give you a reference or incident number for the report.
- Inform them you have asked him not to contact you directly for any reason and to deal with your solicitor (or a third party) when it is necessary.
- Show them photos of the note you left him, that stated you do not want him to contact you directly for any reason.

- You can ask if they would inform him, on your behalf, that they are aware of the situation. No further action should be taken at that time, but the information will be referred to should he attempt to contact or confront you in the future.

I know times in the past when the police in the UK have been happy to do this, and it is within reason and your remit to ask them to do it for you. When they inform him that they are aware of the situation, he may think twice about tracking, stalking, harassing or contacting you.

If he does approach you after that, a call to the police, quoting their reference number will usually stop him from doing it again. Especially if you explain you feel vulnerable, unsafe, scared and at risk.

Remember, all you are trying to do is stop him from contacting you from that point on.

It is imperative to be consistent with your intentions. There is no point in reporting your situation, if you don't report him again, should he try to contact you after you first report him to the authorities. If you are not consistent it may undermine you in their eyes. It is in your own interest to report any future events.

If you don't, and he starts to contact you regularly (which is dangerous to your cause) he may show them previous calls between you and him, where you had not reported them to the police, and he could say he assumed you had changed your mind. In that instance, the police may not take your original report seriously. **Think about this carefully and try not to let your Inner Abuser confuse you with ifs, buts or maybes. Be consistent.**

When I suggest contacting the authorities many women recoil as if it is wrong to even consider it. This can be an indication their subconscious is still regarding their partner's well-being more than their own, and a sign their Inner Abuser still has too much influence on their thoughts.

Let's think of this situation another way ...
Think of a friend or member of your family that you love and care for.

Imagine one day she tells you she has been mentally abused by her partner for a very long time. She tells you he shouts and screams at her for the least little thing, he criticises her cooking, clothes, friends, looks and her family. She says he belittles her, both privately and in front of others. He calls her an idiot, stupid or ugly, and tells her to shut up every time she tries to speak. She tells you she is now living in fear of him, walking on eggshells, and sometimes feels like she's going crazy.

Now, in your mind, add all the things your abusive partner does and says to you.

Imagine *she* is the one suffering all of the abuse that you are.

Now imagine she just told you she has left him and is living in a rented apartment on her own.

After hearing all the abuse he has put her through, would you advise <u>her</u> to ask the police to make a record of the situation in case he appears so that <u>she</u> can feel safer in her new home?

The Inner Abuser thrives on drama, if you diminish the drama in your life, you will diminish your Inner Abuser's influence over you. As this happens, your life will improve too.

ℲJ

Back to the present moment ... right now all you need do is to *consider* notifying the police this could secure long-term protection for you in your new home.

Nothing terrible will happen to him as a result of you making the police aware of your concerns, but it might help you sleep safe and sound at night.

I am lingering on this notion before moving on for a reason; I know it is the single most effective way for you to be safe in your new home. Nothing else will help you more.

It's worth noting that the strength of feeling you have against reporting him, could be a marker of the influence him and your Inner Abuser still have on your thoughts. Somewhere in the back of your mind, are you still concerning yourself with his well-being?

SPECIAL NOTE

If you do report your concerns and then decide to return to your partner, it could weaken your ability to get proper help from the police in the future. Their resolve to bring a mentally abusive individual to justice will be broken if the main witness is not trustworthy or resolute. They are only human.

If you are going to involve the police, wait until you have left, have no intention of returning, and are willing to burn all bridges with your ex. Once you are at that stage, and you show the authorities you are serious about keeping him away from you, they are more likely to give you the support you need to feel safe in your new home.

PREPARATIONS AND PLANS FOR THE DAY YOU LEAVE

In the weeks before you aim to leave, visualise how you want the day to unfold in your head. This will help to put you in a more relaxed frame of mind when the day arrives. As you repeat this, play out anything that may hinder you on the day, and think about solutions to any possible setbacks you might encounter.

If you have confided in a friend or relative who understands the situation, you could ask them to help move the personal possessions you choose to take with you on the day.

Writing out a shortlist of steps to work through on the day will help everything go smoothly.

ON THE DAY

- It is at this point you should switch off your smartphone and remove the SIM, the same goes for any tablet with a SIM. Then put the phone in the signal blocking cover (you should have previously purchased this with cash or on a trusted person's card. Remember not to make electronic payments on your cards for anything that will alert your partner to your plans. He could trace the sale and discover what you purchased).
- Be careful not to take anything with you that is jointly owned, like table lamps, duvets, kitchen utensils or otherwise. Unless of course, you can prove they are exclusively owned by you. Your clothes, shoes, jewellery and all personal items including a passport and personal paperwork, bank statements, etc. are usually classed as owned by you. This is the best approach, it allows you to concentrate on getting yourself out and to a place of safety before there is a chance of him returning unexpectedly.
- Photograph the whole house with a camera, or your friend's smartphone, not yours, because it should be switched off and in the signal blocking pouch by this point in time.
- On leaving, it is imperative that you quickly photograph the condition of the property. Several pictures of each room and the jointly owned items in it are enough.
- Photograph the front and back doors, windows and the outside of the house. This shouldn't take long and the smartphone or camera you use should record the date and time of the photographs.

(The photographs are important and necessary, you only have this one opportunity to do this. Do not discuss these pictures with anyone other than those present at the time you depart.)

- If you are relocating some distance from your abusive partner, do not use the bank/credit cards you had while cohabiting with him. There is a possibility he could find out where you are refuelling or buying groceries, if he has previously hacked your accounts. These cards should be disposed of on the day of departure and any funds removed and deposited in new accounts, with different banks.

(Having to adhere to these recommendations may seem excessive, but they are vital for your safety. I can tell you through experience, that many women have no idea just how devious their DMA partner can be until *after* they try to leave him.)

Do not leave anything to chance, your Inner Abuser may suggest, 'You don't need to bother about this or that, he won't bother chasing you *that* much'. It is dangerous to assume everything will be okay without *you* making sure it is.

- Leave him a SHORT note (or a short letter from your lawyer) saying no more than:
- After much thought you have decided to leave the relationship, you will not return and you do not want him to contact you directly from now on.
- State that you do not want him to come near you from now on. Intimate that your third party or lawyer will contact him in due course for the legal side of the separation.
- Say if he breaks these wishes you will contact the police. (Or you have reported the situation and the information in this note to the police and asked them to create an incident number for you.)

- Ask him to respect your wishes.
- Sign it, date it and leave it in a prominent position in the house, where he will find it as soon as he arrives home.
- Take a photograph of the note itself and another photo of where you left it.

(Remember to ignore any doubt initiated by your Inner Abuser. His abusive nature has made this procedure necessary. All of these actions are designed to safeguard you from further abuse.)

- Be mindful of your Inner Abuser inventing drama on the day you leave, or it may attempt to create a situation where your departure is delayed or fails.
- Be aware of your actions and any delays you impose on yourself on the day.
- Take your clothes, jewellery, personal items and paperwork, and lock the house as you leave.
- If there is anything you have left that is yours alone, make sure you photograph it and if it 'gets damaged', you may be able to claim compensation or have it replaced.
- If there is any garden equipment of great value, ride-on mowers, etc., photograph them as well.

Try not to worry about jointly owned material things left in the house, you can claim for half their value at the time of your departure. Taking too much with you will slow you down and hamper a swift exit.

The prime objective in escaping an abusive relationship is to get *you* away from *him* ... *and* for you to remain away from him with no further direct communication from that moment on.

ARRIVING AT YOUR NEW ACCOMMODATION

After leaving the note and leaving the premises, you should not use any electronic equipment or bank/credit card that you owned previously, they are traceable by GPS or at the point of any purchase you make with the cards.

It is illegal for him to track you *without your consent*, however, it is unlikely this will stop him from trying. It's a law that is not enforced unless it is reported (*in the UK*).

₪

Programme his known numbers into your new phone and block them. If you get a call from any unknown numbers, **do not** answer them, if anyone wants to contact you they should leave a message on your voicemail. If you do get harassed by multiple unknown numbers, you can always block them too. Anyone that needs to contact you legitimately will find a way. Make a note of any unknown numbers that call, without leaving a voicemail.

If you have informed the authorities about your situation, and he does attempt to contact you, ask them to record the call details and explain that you do not know how he got the number. They will take the appropriate action. This may be all you need to stop him from trying to communicate with you directly again.

As a last resort, you can always dispose of the new SIM and replace it with another new one. They cost very little, and if you have stored your contacts in your phone instead of the SIM you can tell the people you trust your new number. Make sure your number is withheld before making calls with the new SIM card.

Some texting apps will not withhold your number so be careful you don't inadvertently send your number with the text.

Texting may show your number, so take note. If in doubt, send a message to a trusted friend, to check if the number is sent along with the text.

If you leave a note asking him not to try to contact you and he tries to, he has ignored it and disrespected your wishes. This is another indication he doesn't care about what you want, and only about what he wants.

₪

In the first few months after leaving you may have to deal with other people's Inner Abuser too. This may become apparent when they try to give you advice. They may be upset at your decision to leave, but it might be because it impacts them, not you, and their Inner Abuser may try to address that. They may even question why you left without telling him you were going.

If they are sceptical, reassure them you are sure of what you are doing and ask them to remain patient, while the situation develops.

When speaking with friends or family, it's the best policy not to share any evidence you have and may use during any legal settlements.

₪

If your ex manages to find his way to your door offering gifts, do not open the door and do not accept any gifts. If he leaves any gifts outside your door photograph them before disposing of them. My advice is not to put flowers in water or eat any chocolates. Nor would I wear any clothes or jewellery. Try to imagine that they don't exist, and find a way to dispose of them. You do not want to take any comfort from anything he leaves, it will work against your determination to overcome the effects of DMA in your subconscious.

To the uninitiated, gifts may make him look more sincere, however apologising with bunches of flowers or elaborate handouts, is simply another form of emotional abuse when coming from these individuals.

If he leaves anything at your door as an 'apology' take pictures of it and any apologetic notes accompanying it. However tempting it may be, you should pass them on or dispose of them. Maybe you could give them to a friend or neighbour, but don't keep them, they will remind you of him every time you lay eyes on them, so dispose of them, without exception. Apologies and promises are a tactic used by an abuser to confuse their partner's mind. These gifts are his Trojan Horses, don't allow them past your defences.

If he manages to contact you after you leave, record it and back it up on other devices. It could make it easier to prove his harassment if others question your version of the situation.

Those doubting the position you take during all of this may rethink if you give them some proof of his abuse or harassment. Some may not though, so don't waste valuable energy trying to convince them, if early attempts fail. Most people's ideas will change over time and if you realise that to begin with, it makes it all easier to deal with. If some choose to take his side, distance yourself from their negativity, it's important for your recovery.

It may be difficult at first, but as you grow stronger, losing some people's friendships will not seem such a big deal. You may even come to realise losing them was a blessing in disguise. If they see their opinion as more important than your happiness in life, then they may not be who you need for support going forward anyway.

Choosing to avoid certain people who do not have your best interests at heart, is part of the process to overcome mental abuse as quickly as possible. Criticism may not only be aimed at you from your ex, it could, even inadvertently, come from others you may have expected more from. If this happens, it can be a good thing. There is no point in draining your energy trying to appease them, respect yourself first, put your needs ahead of theirs, avoid them where possible, tolerate them when necessary, and try not to waste good energy on needless conversation. Remember, you are allowed to choose what is best for you in your life, it may be that his mental abuse has diminished your ability to see your self-worth. In the act of leaving him, you have shown your intent to reverse that influence.

You might expect most people to be sympathetic to you, but try not to get upset if some of them let you down. There is no way of knowing what's really on their mind if they don't give you the support you expected. There may even be those that try to sabotage your separation, not because it is good for you but because it makes things easier for them. People that enjoyed your company as a couple could be disappointed that the dynamics have changed, and for their own sake, would prefer you got back together.

As a result, they may prefer their status quo to continue and try to convince you he wasn't that bad. That may be okay for them, but they were not the ones he was abusing, you were. It is better knowing certain people may not be the ideal company for a while after you leave. Use your intuition and be aware of who you choose to be around.

As time passes, most people who genuinely care about your happiness will accept your new status.

Know in your heart that you are heading towards a better life, keep using this book to stay strong, and your authentic friends should continue to support you.

BEGINNING A NEW LIFE IN YOUR NEW HOME

- It's a good idea to put a single (at least) CCTV camera with a microphone at your new front door. They are quite cheap and easy to install nowadays. It's a great way to record evidence if your ex-partner finds his way to your new home.
- Most can be linked to a smartphone too. They will record for a set period when any movement is detected.
- If, as advised, you don't use a smartphone for the first few months (because they are too easy to track), you may need to ask someone you have confided in to link it to their smart phone, if you are both happy that they will get alerts when anyone turns up at your door.
- If your ex turns up, they can record the event as evidence for the police, or your lawyer.
- It could also allow you to prove to those around you that he was at your door against your wishes.
- The recording will destroy any denial from him, that he was there.

Using these devices sends a clear message to your abuser … **You want him out of your life**. It also shows the authorities and your friends and family that you are serious and resolute about the separation.

If you are staying with friends, you will need to discuss the possibility that he may turn up, uninvited, and how best to handle it. You may even want to act it out between you. This is a great way of pre-programming you and them in the event of him appearing at the door. Convince them it is much better to prepare for this than end up panicking if he does make an appearance without prior warning. If in doubt, don't open the door, and phone the police.

BE PREPARED FOR YOUR PARTNER TRYING TO FIND YOU
… not because he loves you, but because he thinks he 'owns' you.

Don't be fooled into a false sense of security, if he uses the 'thirty days no contact' rule. It's a simple reverse psychology technique to trick you into getting in touch with him out of some subconscious concern. If you make that mistake, he is sure to save it on his phone as evidence to others that, 'you contacted him, and he didn't contact you'. In one weak moment, you could undo **ALL** of your good work to get this far. Your side of the argument will melt away if you are the one to make the first contact after the separation.

This situation can be used to your advantage though.

No contact with your abuser is the best way to help you move on, so if he uses the, 'thirty days no contact' rule, it will give you some time to prepare for your new life going forward (if he uses it). Look at this lack of intrusion from him as one of the best things that could happen to you.
I assure you, it is.

You may not be able to stop him from manipulating other people's thoughts, but you can stop him from manipulating yours.

Try to remind yourself that this is your new life, he is no longer a part of it, try to stop yourself whenever he has re-entered your mind. Focus on something uplifting to get your mind going in another direction.

There is a small exercise you can use whenever you find yourself thinking about him … when he creeps back into your thoughts, just say: STOP, THESE THOUGHTS DO NOT SERVE ME, out loud if possible, and replace thoughts about him with thoughts about you, for example:

- If you find yourself thinking 'I wonder how he's doing', replace it with, 'How am I doing, what can I do right now to make **me** feel better?'
- If you find yourself thinking, 'I wonder where he is?', replace it with, 'What am I enjoying about where I am right now?' or 'Where can I go right now, that will make **me** feel good?'.

Get into the way of focusing on things that will make **you** feel better any time he appears in your thoughts. Don't beat yourself up, this is a process that you will win, but it takes practice. Write this small exercise down and use it as often as you can.

These are your thoughts, **you** have the power to choose what you think about, but it takes time to train your Authentic Self to take control. You won't always have to put so much effort into it, you will soon be focusing on yourself and not him, naturally, straight from your subconscious mind.

TO RECAP THE FIRST FEW DAYS AND WEEKS AFTER LEAVING:

- Immerse yourself in the mental exercises of Part 2.
- Always consider **your** safety first (mentally as well as physically).
- Use your lawyer for any legal contact with your ex.
- Use a third party you trust as a contact for other matters. Someone who understands his abusive nature. They only discuss a single pre-agreed subject. This should always be by email or text so that they, and you, have a record of it. If he makes any attempt to discuss anything else (in particular his feelings) they must remind him of the reason for the email or text.

- Only as a last resort or in an emergency should there be a phone call. Notify him in writing, through your third party or lawyer, that in an emergency he must leave a voicemail as the call will not be answered. Ask your third party if they would install a free call recording app on their phone. That way they can record any conversation they have with him after he leaves a voicemail message.
- Remind them to pre-arrange any calls with him by text and **never** answer any calls from him other than at already prearranged times. It is **very important** to set these boundaries. He will try to flaunt them and you (and your third party) must be strong.
- Try to limit the third party contact to emails, in this way you have proof of exactly what he says in writing.
- His spoken words are the most dangerous to you and others, avoiding them and his voice is for everyone's safety and benefit.
- Using only written contact gives you, and your go-between, the chance to discuss any response to him before making it.
- After leaving him do not use any of your old communication devices, numbers or email addresses. (If necessary, only check incoming mail to old email addresses, NEVER use them to send anything after you have left him), he may have access to them that you are unaware of.
- Set up new devices, new SIM cards, new phone numbers and new email addresses.
- Block his number on these devices.
- Block his emails on your old email addresses.
- Do not answer any new calls from numbers you do not know.
- Do not open any emails when you do not recognise the sender (ask a friend to do this if you are not sure, you mustn't be tempted to read anything he sends you directly, through any means).

- REMEMBER, mental abuse is an attack on your mind, your thoughts, emotions and feelings. He does this through communication, no communication equals no further mental abuse.
- Tell him to contact your lawyer in the case of an 'emergency'. (Remember, in life, there are very few situations where communication is needed instantly.)
- Ask anyone who may call you, to leave a voicemail if they don't get you.
- Inform those that you trust with your new contact details that on NO account should they give your ex your new details.
- Consider a cheap single-camera CCTV device at your new front door.
- Ask to link it to your trusted confidant's smartphone/s.
- Remind yourself, that he may use the 'thirty-day no contact rule' to trick you into contacting him, don't fall for it. Any period when you do not hear from him or 'of him' is extremely beneficial to your recovery from DMA.
- Continue to immerse yourself in the mental exercises in Part 2 of this book.
- Keep reminding yourself, that with emotional abusers, **no** contact is always the best way for your safety and recovery.
- Ask anyone you give contact details to, to keep them hidden from anyone else, even their family. He may try to convince their husband (or wife), to divulge your whereabouts or phone number. (I heard of an abuser pretending their child had been in an accident while in his care and he needed to contact her immediately … the accident was a lie.)
- For the first few months, the fewer people who have your details the better.

- If possible only give your details to one confidant and ask everyone else to contact you through them. In this way, only one person will have to keep your details secure.
- While you may have to go to work, and he will know where that is, when possible, stay inside for lunch and if you go out, try to be with a colleague that is likely to support you in the event he turns up.
- MAKE IT A LEGAL SEPARATION IN THE EYES OF THE LAW IN YOUR COUNTRY, seek legal advice on how to do this under your local laws. It will help if he attempts to accost or harass you.

Your Inner Abuser will try to convince you a lot of this is unnecessary, so consider these possibilities:

1. You follow all the guidelines above, and he tries to contact you. But, because you are mentally and physically prepared for that, you repel the attempt unreservedly through lawyers, your confidants or the authorities to ensure he doesn't do it again. **You win.**

2. You follow the guidelines and he never contacts you directly again. **You win.**

3. You don't follow these guidelines and he never contacts you directly again. **You win.**

OR

4. You don't follow the guidelines, and he contacts you, you are unprepared and succumb to his promises or threats. You move back in with him. **You lose.**

5. You don't follow the guidelines, and you contact him. He shows everyone the details he has saved on his phone, and you lose all credibility with the police and those around you. You succumb to his promises or threats and return to live with him. **You lose.**

6. You don't follow the guidelines, you don't make a plan, you don't

bother using a lawyer or third party, you succumb to his words of promise or threat and move back in with him. **You lose.**

7. If you don't make a plan, choose a confidant, a lawyer or inform the authorities.

If you are not mentally or physically prepared for this.

If you return to cohabit with him, back where you started.

If the abuse is worse in the future.

You lose.

If you choose not to follow the guidance in this book you could be in greater danger of slipping back into the relationship again, like most mentally abused women do.

They lost.

The sole purpose of this book is to help all women. So if everyone follows the guidelines ...

We might all win.

₪

Up until now millions of women around the world have not been able to break free from their abusive partner due to the influence of his DMA on their thoughts, emotions and feelings. Most of them were simply not aware of the changes his abuse had on their thought processes or their ability to see the truth in their predicament.

Up until now, most women have had no proper guidance to understand that their thoughts have been corrupted by their partner's DMA, and that is the very reason they feel so confused about their life.

- Up until now, it has only been researchers and academics who have been aware that the part of the mind I call the 'Inner Abuser' exists.

- Up until now, most women have never heard of the Inner Abuser.
- By reading this book **you** now know the Inner Abuser exists.
- For the first time, **you** can become aware of the Inner Abuser's influence.
- Now, for the first time, you can start to challenge the thoughts produced by your Inner Abuse, as a result of DMA.
- Now you can understand why your mind has been working against you.
- Now you can use this book to reverse the effects DMA has had on you.
- Now you are aware it was the Inner Abuser's decisions in the past that created your present situation.
- Now you know that if you want to change the present situation you must not allow that part of your mind to make any more big decisions.
- Now you know it has been a strong influence on your mind and you can begin to overcome the decisions it has been controlling if you want to make better choices for your future.

Now you know the Inner Abuser is to blame for the choices you made in the past. By working with this book you have an opportunity to reject any idea you are a 'victim' of this DMA situation or your partner. Now you realise you have the power in yourself, to strengthen your mind, and take back control of your life.

You are ready to begin using the mental exercises that will help you overcome your Inner Abuser's influence and reverse the effects DMA has had on your life.

REMEMBER, mental abuse is an attack on your mind, your thoughts, emotions and feelings. He does this through communication, no communication equals no further mental abuse.

CHAPTER 10

GETTING READY TO START THE MENTAL EXERCISES

You should only begin these exercises once you fully understand Part 1 of the book, re-read it if necessary, while remembering to stop along the way when you see this sign, ⌘ to think about what you have just read. Acknowledging the existence of the Inner Abuser is paramount to your level of success with this book. There is no quick way to overcome DMA if you don't understand the main reason it was able to affect your thoughts and the way you see the world. Even if you are unaware of the changes since you met your abusive partner.

The Inner Abuser can also be known as a part of the 'Ego', 'The Inner Chimp' or 'The Black Wolf'. Regardless of how it is described in different cultures around the world, the fact is, that this 'self-sabotaging entity' exists in all of us.

Modern neuroscience, traditional psychology, ancient proverbs and old sayings all acknowledge the existence of this part of our mind, and how it works against us. When we are exposed to mental and emotional abuse it gets stronger and by creating unhelpful beliefs, it enslaves us. It can convince you there is no way out of a DMA situation, and it will invent reasons and excuses to lock you in an abusive relationship.

It is well known that people under stress make bad decisions, this is when the Inner Abuser takes control and it uses your partner's mental abuse to assist it. It feeds on the drama created by daily emotional abuse and convinces you that you're trapped in the situation with no way out.

The first thing to do to overcome DMA is to free your mind.

You have the power in you to beat DMA properly and to have a happier life from this moment on, but rushing through this book, without fully understanding what you are reading is not the way to achieve that. The way to beat DMA *faster* is to read this book *slower*, that is why you see the symbol ₪ when it is '*time to stop and think about what you have just read*'.

Reading quickly is not going to help you beat DMA, slowing down to fully understand the information here, and practising these exercises repeatedly will. This way of reprogramming your mind can deal with your situation effectively, but will only work if it is followed correctly. Take a moment to realise this is to help you beat the long-term effects DMA has caused, so try to be patient. You are about to begin reprogramming your mind to default to positive thoughts in any situation.

It is mental abuse, abuse of the mind, and the mind is the first place to reverse the damage DMA has caused.

₪

After reading the introduction to your Inner Abuser and the list of abuse, you should know by now if you are in a DMA relationship or not. But the Inner Abuser still has its trump card left to play … 'love'. When all the attempts to manipulate your mind have failed, it will try to convince you that, you still love your abuser … and you really don't want to leave him.

Only your 'Authentic Self' will know if this is true, but you may have to spend some time contemplating if the 'love' is real, or just your Inner Abuser trying to convince you it is.

It's your Inner Abuser against your Authentic Self, the black wolf against the white wolf, the chimp mind versus the human mind.
Who will win?
As always, it will be … **The One you Feed.**

Ask yourself, 'How can this be love, who would love someone that has abused them so much?'

Is it love?

Or is it another covert trick distorting the way you 'feel' after so much mental abuse.

What is love?

You need to know what love really is, before allowing your Inner Abuser to use it against you.

Mental abuse is brainwashing, it doesn't mean you are a zombie and entirely controlled by your abusive partner, you still function as a separate thinking being, but you only have free will over the things your DMA partner isn't bothered about controlling …

… he's quite happy for you to take the kids to school, dress them, feed them and keep them clean and healthy … he might be quite happy for you to carry out your daily chores without too much interference from him. You might feel quite normal driving, commuting or interacting with others …

But … the areas of your life your partner wants to control, the way you think, the way you act and the way you feel in those moments, he does control. Even if you are not aware of it.

If you stop to think about it, you may realise that in certain situations, the way you act, what you say, what you do and how you feel are all influenced by him and usually for his benefit. When you find yourself defending him against any suggestion of abuse from others, you might just realise, deep down, he is manipulating you. If you catch yourself saying things you know are not true, just to cover up for him, you may realise, you're doing it for his benefit, even when he's not around and when he doesn't deserve it.

DMA brainwashing is real. Take some time to imagine he simply did not exist (not that he has died, but that he simply vanished and does not exist, he never has, but everything else remains the same).

Think about it, and ask yourself, 'How would I act differently right now?'

Would you be more confident?

Would you be more sociable?

Would you be happier?

He does not exist, so if you thought about any of these questions and he was any part of the answer, you are not visualising the situation properly. He doesn't exist, he never has, how do you feel?

Are you still thinking about him?

Think about yourself, you are single, you can do anything you want, go anywhere you want, experience anything you want, whenever you want to.

This exercise might help you to recognise he has a bigger influence on your life and on your ability to be free than you realised up until now.

₪

Eventually, as he continues to manipulate your mind, you may be convinced that you 'love' him. Even when your situation becomes very dangerous, and your fear of him is complete, your Inner Abuser can still convince you that you 'still love him' and you don't really want to leave him.

The Inner Abuser will encourage you to tell others you 'still love him' because it is difficult for them to argue against how you 'feel' and who you 'love'.

After all, how could they know how you actually 'feel'?

And if this is an excuse you are hiding behind right now, do *you* know how you actually 'feel'?

Are *you* being honest with yourself? Or is your Inner Abuser answering for you, to keep you in a relationship that will only become worse as time goes by?

The use of love is the Inner Abuser's best argument, and one it will try to convince you is real. Once it does, it will encourage you to use love as an excuse, the real reason why you cannot leave him. Others can find it hard to get past your declaration of love when trying to convince you to leave an abusive partner.

If there's a possibility you may be using love as an excuse to justify putting up with mental abuse think about this scenario …

₪

If you told someone about your abusive partner and they advised you to get away from him, your Inner Abuser is still capable of playing its ace. Even after describing all the abuse in detail, you may still find yourself trying to end the conversation by saying, 'I can't leave him, I know you think this is crazy after all I've told you, but I still love him.'

However, thinking about someone all the time is not necessarily driven by 'love'.

Just because you are frightened of being on your own, it doesn't necessarily mean you 'love' *him*. Nor does it mean you can't live without *him*.

Just because you are scared of leaving your partner, it doesn't necessarily mean you still 'love' him …

… there is much that could be added to this list, and all of it is based on fear, created by his DMA and your Inner Abuser.

Certain compelling feelings to stay with him may manifest in your mind as love, when in fact it is the domestic relationship equivalent of Stockholm syndrome. A recognised psychological effect on the human mind that is based on fear of the individuals who are holding you against your will. Eventually, there comes a time when you sympathise with or defend the person or people responsible for your capture, kidnapping or control.

Be careful if you feel the urge to use the word 'love' when you discuss your situation with others. If you tell them you can't leave him because you still 'love' him, it could curtail their determination and ability to help you. They may feel they can't continue to put forward much of a case for leaving, if you convince them you still 'love' him.

So do you? Do you really?

Hopefully, that idea is long gone, but if you are contemplating it, ask yourself again, 'how could I have a love for someone that treats me so badly and manipulates my mind?'
Ask yourself this too, 'Is it possible I have been brainwashed into this ideology?'
Is it possible, not is it a fact, is it *possible*?

It *is* possible.

The exercises in Part 2 will help diminish any false feelings of 'love', and in time, they will disappear completely. DMA and your Inner Abuser can conceal the reality of a situation, and they mess with your mind enough to make you remain in a relationship with an abusive man.

Love is many things, but it is not the 'feeling' you get for someone who abuses you, that feeling is a product of his abuse and will decrease if you use this book correctly. It will fade away as you regain the ability to recognise what is real and what is imagined (through the influence of DMA) in your life.

I remember a case of serious mental abuse, when I asked the woman, 'What is the one thing you would like to have in your life from now on?', and she said, 'Happiness'.

It's not possible to be in a DMA relationship and be genuinely happy. Your Inner Abuser may manage to convince you that 'It's not that bad' and 'he isn't abusive all the time', but it will not be able to convince you that you are genuinely happy, or that you could ever be happy while in that relationship.

This book is designed to help you find that happiness in the future, and through that happiness, discover true love and not that 'feeling' you have for someone who abuses your mind and manipulates your thoughts.

Ask yourself these questions:
- Do **you** genuinely believe you could be in 'love' with someone that is so cruel to you?
- How could **you** actually 'love' someone who has abused you so much that you're no longer sure what love is anymore?
- Would anyone who genuinely loves *you* treat you this way?

The human mind defers us to the people and places we are familiar with, even when they are detrimental to our mental and sometimes physical health. We crave the familiar even when it is hurtful and abusive. This phenomenon assisted by the Inner Abuser is part of the reason we find it hard to leave. These feelings we have toward a mentally abusive individual are rarely based on true love, but simply on the perverse way the human mind works in certain circumstances. If we choose to reverse these problems on a conscious level, we can. It only takes two things:

- recognising that your present situation will never allow you to have a happy life
- recognising you have the ability in you, to change it.

How many abused women are living with 'familiar' surroundings, instead of a happy life?
Can being emotionally abused by your partner forever, be a happy life?

Are your 'familiar' surroundings creating a happy life for you?

Do you think, being with a mentally abusive partner (who is only going to become more abusive in time) is really where **you** should be for the rest of your life?

₪

If you have already escaped your abusive partner in the physical sense, using this book will help you clear any lingering psychological effects that mental abuse planted in the back of your mind. They need to be removed to be completely free again and to completely love someone once more.

Using this book will change your mind, literally. Even if you are fearful at this moment in time, you can soon feel courage and confidence again. Imagine what it would be like to be fearless … seriously, imagine how you would feel if you were afraid of nothing. You may have lost some self-belief recently, but you won't have lost your imagination, and it's important to use it. What would it feel like to you, to be fearless?

₪

If you find yourself trying to read on without taking this time out to do some visualisation, stop right now, take some time out and imagine a life without fear. This little exercise is much more important than you may be aware of at this very moment in time.

₪

If you use this book properly, you should begin to see your life changing for the better. Your inner strength will start returning even if you believed it was gone for good. If you don't use it properly, it will always be 'just another book', a collection of words and recommendations you didn't make the effort to follow or didn't believe in.

It could remain, just another book, but the power is not in the book, the power is in **you**, and if **you do** follow the recommendations properly, what you discover in these pages can help to change your life.

Just as we all need some daily exercise to keep the body fit and healthy, we also need daily mental exercise to keep the mind healthy too. If your mind has been affected by DMA, these exercises are designed to reverse the damage it has done.

I recall a rather tragic case, when a woman was transformed, almost overnight, using the continuous repetition of one of the exercises you are about to learn. After repeating this single exercise over and over for about an hour, and then several more times that same night, she was literally, like a new woman, the very next day.

However, even though she attributed her miraculous transformation to this exercise, she stopped using it regularly soon after! She stopped taking the twenty minutes a day to exercise her mind and within a week or two, returned to the DMA partner she had tried so hard to escape. If you don't continue to exercise your mind every day, you will be in real danger of reverting to the world your Inner Abuser created for you. The world of domestic mental abuse.

Resistance to change is one of the biggest challenges to overcome.

Over the next few weeks you must stay vigilant to recognise any resistance to your new routine of daily mental exercises. Interference from your Inner Abuser could hamper your progress at any time and it is now up to you to make sure nothing gets in the way of practising these exercises daily.

Do you remember this affirmation from earlier in the book? …

I WANT THIS, I WANT TO CHANGE

You can use it now, to encourage you to keep this new habit going. You have to 'WANT THIS' new regime of daily mental exercises.
Why?

Because this is one of the most powerful ways to overcome the effects DMA has on your subconscious mind.

You have to 'WANT THIS CHANGE', to overcome DMA.

₪

If you are feeling deflated at the idea of having to keep up these mindful exercises every day, think about this:

Imagine you joined a gym and worked hard to tone your body up. Imagine at the end of the year you were pleased with the results. Now imagine what would happen if you stopped going to the gym, and stopped maintaining that new fit 'you'. How long would it be before you started recognising your 'old self' in the mirror again?

The mind is no different from the body. If you don't maintain the new mind this book can help you create, it won't be long before you start to recognise the influences of the Inner Abuser and your old mind creeping back into your life.

The old mind, and the decisions it made, led you to your present situation.
The new mind will repair all the damage that the old one caused.
What mind you follow in the future, is in your hands.

Your new mind will be able to deal with life's difficulties, and it will also overcome the obstacles that DMA created in your old mind. The old mind has been run by your Inner Abuser and fuelled by DMA. Fear, guilt and shame are products of this old mind.

₪

By now, you should be left with no doubt that your partner's mental abuse has caused these emotions in recent times. If you are still doubting if your Inner Abuser and DMA are responsible for the way you are feeling right now, you may have to read Part 1 again. When you are reading, it's easy to miss a vital piece of the jigsaw if other thoughts distract you, even momentarily. Your eyes may continue to skim over the pages, but you're not taking in what you read. Without being aware of it, you may be thinking about something else, and you miss an essential message that page contains.

₪

You know those 'feelings' of dread, despair or danger that appear as if from nowhere and with no apparent reason? As you work with these exercises, they will fade away, replaced by new, more positive thoughts and feelings of optimism and enthusiasm for life.

Your partner repeated his abuse over and over again for a reason. He was programming your subconscious bit by bit each time he repeated the same words and actions. He was slowly eroding your mind's natural ability to defend itself from his continued mental abuse. Repetition is one of the main reasons DMA is so successful at literally changing someone's mind.

The exercises in this book are designed to reverse these changes, but just like your partner's repetition of cruel words and phrases, you need to be prepared to do them over and over again, daily. Your Inner Abuser may try to tell you that these exercises are not worth it, but when the alternative is the ever downward spiralling life with a mental abuser, they are.

- The more you repeat the exercises the quicker you can expect results.
- They won't work if you don't do them. (How could they?)
- They won't have any long-lasting effect if you only do them a handful of times. (Compare it to physical exercise, it also needs a lot of repetition to see positive results.)
- They will only work properly if you make them part of your life, just as DMA has been part of your life for so long.
- This book will only work if you stick closely to the recommendations in it.
- **Transformation of your mind will happen, but only if you work with the book regularly and continue to do so in the long term.**

If your Inner Abuser is still strong enough to create a doubt in your mind that these exercises can change your life so much, think about it this way: You will never really know how effective they can be, without actually following the course. The only thing you can truly predict is if you decide to do nothing … nothing will happen.

If you are finding it hard to believe that the repetition of some simple exercises can make any difference in your life, ask yourself …

- 'Even though I can't believe this will work as it all seems too simple, why don't I at least try?'
- 'It isn't even costing me money, so why wouldn't I just try it?'
- 'If it only costs me time, and not even much of that, what is holding me back?'
- 'If I want a happy future free from DMA and the way it makes me feel, why don't I just commit to this course?'
- Why does it feel so difficult to commit to something promising me so much?'

Of course, the answer to all of these questions is that your Inner Abuser's influence on your mind is still very strong … for the moment, at least.

₪

If you feel any negativity towards this book, it isn't your Authentic Self that is creating that feeling, it's your subconscious and your Inner Abuser.
Try to concentrate on this …
YOU … Have to want a new life free of DMA more than anything.
YOU … Have to want this new happier life more than anything.
YOU … Have to want to do these exercises over and over again.
YOU … Have to be ready to do what it takes to achieve all of this …
… that's when this book can deliver.

₪

I know of no adverse effects from doing the exercises in this book, at the very worst, if you do not stick to the programme properly, you won't feel the benefits that can be achieved. However, if you follow the exercises the way they are set out and explained, your mind will become more positive each time you do them. You may not notice much at first, because it's the repetition of these exercises that cause the changes to take place. Learning the actual exercises is easy, it is the cumulative effects of the REPETITIVE PROCESS that will create the changes in your mind and your life. The more you do the exercises, the quicker these changes will happen.

Have faith in yourself and your ability to beat DMA completely. Look forward to a brighter future, because you are about to create a stronger mind to get you there, and keep you there.

We all need to begin this course of exercises in the best possible state of mind, and if the first half of the book has done its job, you should be feeling more optimistic about changing your life for the better. Ideally, by now, your diet contains less of the food that can cause a downward spiral in our emotions and more of the mood-enhancing food that helps to raise our vibrations. It's just one of the lifestyle changes that will help you believe in yourself a little bit more, but everything you have read up until now should have helped in some way, to set you up for these exercises.

Let's go.

CHAPTER 11

A COURSE OF SIMPLE BUT POWERFUL EXERCISES DESIGNED TO GENTLY REVERSE THE PSYCHOLOGICAL EFFECTS CAUSED BY DMA

A few years ago I met up with an old friend I hadn't seen for many years. He was going through some hard times, but it was obvious listening to him, that he was creating most of the misfortune himself. I told him, I had discovered how to create amazing transformations in my life, just by using certain techniques to transform my mind. I learned how to decrease my stress, and increase my happiness and my finances. He became very interested in the conversation and asked if I could help him do the same.

The advice I gave him was similar, in some respects, to the exercises you are about to begin in this book. I told him my research showed these exercises worked every time and with everyone that used them properly … without exception. He had to repeat particular mental exercises as often as possible, daily, until the things he wanted started to materialise. It was that simple.

Before we parted I said to him, 'For anything on the outside to change, you have to change the inside first, your mind. Remember, you have to repeat these exercises regularly for anything to change. If you don't do them, they don't work. Simple as that. Do not stop, and you will get what you want, the more you work with them the sooner this will happen.'

Many months later I made a point of contacting him to see how he was doing and asked, 'How's life? Have the exercises been working for you? Did you get what you wanted?'

Knowing him well enough I wasn't surprised when he said, 'No, they didn't work, so I stopped doing them.'

He sounded quite indignant as if it was my fault he hadn't achieved his goal! He was a victim of his Inner Abuser, and he simply didn't want these changes to happen **enough** to overcome the influence of his Inner Abuser. You have to want something badly enough in your mind before you can make it happen in reality and you must not give up until you see the changes happen in your physical world.

You have the power within your mind to break the mentality DMA and your Inner Abuser have created. How much do you want to do that?

₪

My friend's Inner Abuser convinced him that he should have achieved his desires by a certain time and when that didn't happen he just stopped. Even though he had no prior knowledge of the massive success attributed to these techniques, he was persuaded by his Inner Abuser to stop. It convinced him to believe he knew better than me, without ever having studied or researched the subject matter himself. Even after I told him this takes time, and it takes a different length of time for everyone. Even after being told it *always* works, he decided to stop. He just didn't want it **enough**.

**Remember Henry Ford again,
'Whether you think you can or you think you can't, you're probably right.'**

The truth was, regardless of what my friend said, deep down he didn't want to achieve his goals enough. Over the years he had become accustomed to apathy and failure. It sort of felt 'right' to him to struggle through life because that's what he was used to.

If he told me he didn't like the jacket he was wearing, and I offered him a better one, he would probably keep wearing the old one anyway. Even though he said he didn't like it, he would keep wearing it, because it was familiar to him. The human mind doesn't like change. We profess to want something to change and then when we are given the opportunity, we make reasons and excuses why we can't accept what we wanted so much.

Don't let your mind trick you into remaining with an abusive partner just because he is familiar to you. It is up to you to decide you want a new life enough so that you commit to these mental exercises and never stop doing them, even when you start experiencing the rewards for the effort you put into practising them every day.

Familiarity is a tool used by our Inner Abuser to imprison us in situations that we don't even like. The Inner Abuser creates fear of anything new in our subconscious. The old saying, 'nobody likes change' is based on this. Coming out of our comfort zone is never easy, even when the comfort zone is in a relationship with an abusive partner. Even when that 'comfort zone' is a life of abuse. If you choose to be with someone just because they are familiar to you, by default, **you are also choosing to continue to be abused by them**.

Remind yourself that fear of change is natural, but it's quite unnatural to continue being abused in a relationship, on the premise that you feel apprehensive about a change in your life. DMA creates doubt and fear, so apprehension is not unnatural. You have to be aware of the source of these unwanted feelings and ignore them.

Our Inner Abuser will never completely leave us, but by becoming more vigilant, we can override its influence, whenever we recognise its presence.

If you won't try to change your situation yourself, no one else can. You might remain a virtual slave to your Inner Abuser and your DMA partner for life.

I know you don't want that, but you have to initiate the change yourself. It is you that has to want this change, and want the uncomfortable feeling you will experience at first. Deep down, **you**

know that uncomfortable feeling will pass and it will be replaced by joy and happiness as part of a better life in the future.

So, if you truly want to change your situation you have to want to change, by telling yourself over and over, 'I want this, I really want this and I am not stopping these exercises, ever, I want to change my life forever.'

Having the desire to do the exercises is as important as the exercises themselves.

There's a little affirmation that is powerful and can be used to keep you motivated:

I want to do these exercises,
I want to do these exercises every day,
I know they will reverse the effects of DMA.

₪

My friend didn't know it at the time, but I gave him the equivalent of a winning lottery ticket, that would soon come up if he kept repeating the techniques I told him to use.

Sadly, after a few weeks, his Inner Abuser convinced him the techniques would never work, it convinced him he knew better than me, that he was right and I was wrong. So he stopped using the exercises and at that point, the possibility of his lottery win stopped too.

When I explained his Inner Abuser had stopped him from using the techniques before they had a chance to work, he wouldn't believe it. In his mind, it was nonsense, and they didn't work. His Inner Abuser is still running his mind to this day, and he still finds life a struggle. This is an example of how crucial it is to recognise the Inner Abuser, and the influence it can have on our life and our happiness.

Take a lesson from my friend, don't allow your Inner Abuser to continue forever making the wrong decisions in your life.

My friend made no real effort to allow these techniques to start working before he stopped trying. Before you begin these exercises, be realistic about the time it will take until you become aware that there are positive changes to your mindset appearing. You might not feel anything for a few weeks, or you might just feel a little calmer, a little more in control, or a tiny bit more optimistic about the future. Even if you feel nothing at all, these exercises will be working at a subconscious level. The 'roots' of change will be growing, even if you don't see the 'shoots' on the surface at the same time. If you decide to stop feeding these 'roots' with mental exercises, they will die, and you will soon lose the benefits of any work that you already put in.

We are never aware of plants growing beneath the surface before the shoots appear above the ground, but the plants are still working hard, pushing through the soil to reach the air and the sunshine above.

This is exactly the way these exercises work at first. They have to get a grip, develop and then appear in the form of positive changes to your mindset, so try to ignore any ideas that they are not working, just because you can't see any changes at first. The changes will come, all you need to do is have faith and continue to do the work. If you are impatient for change, do them more frequently, and concentrate on them as you do them.

> No one can lose weight just by *reading* a 'Diet Book'.
> *Reading* the book won't help.
> You have to *follow the advice i*n it if you want to lose weight.
> No one can make a meal, just by *reading* a 'Recipe Book'.
> *Reading* the book won't help.

You have to *follow the advice* in it if you want to make the meal.
No one can change their life, just by *reading* 'This Book'.
Reading the book won't help.
You have to *follow the advice* in it if you want to change your life.

It's that simple.

The exercises don't make many references to DMA, no constant reminder of your present situation or your DMA partner. They work on a subconscious level, they don't fight DMA directly, they gradually strengthen your mind, and as that happens your Inner Abuser's influence diminishes. You do not focus on your partner or his abuse while doing them, in fact, it is the exact opposite, you focus on yourself, and a new future.

IT MIGHT HELP TO COMPARE THESE TWO SITUATIONS

Here, the standard print describes what can happen to your physical body and **the bold print describes what can happen to your mind**:

Imagine you begin to spend more and more of your time on the couch watching TV, unaware that your muscles and your stamina are fading away as the months go by.

Imagine as you spend more and more time with your partner, unaware his mental abuse is affecting your mind, and your self-confidence is slowly fading away as the months go by.

A day comes when you realise you are overweight and unfit, so you decide you are going to run a marathon.

A day comes when you realise your mind has been affected by mental abuse, so you decide to work with this book.

On day one of your new regime, you get off the couch and walk to the end of your street. That's all you can manage and at the end of the day, nothing in your body feels different.

On day one, you follow the first exercise in the book, and nothing in your mind feels different.

You walk every day for a week. Then the following week, you do it twice a day.

You practise the first mental exercise every day for a week, the following week you add the second exercise and do them both more often each day.

The week after that you start to jog instead of walk.

The week after that you add another mental exercise and repeat them regularly.

The week after that you jog twice as far ... as you begin to feel physically stronger.

The week after that you add another mental technique ... as your mind begins to feel stronger.

One day, you look in the mirror and recognise you have lost some weight and you look more toned.

One day, you look into your eyes in the mirror knowing you are more positive, self-assured and less fearful.

You didn't notice your body transforming daily, but the effects of your running are obvious now.

You didn't notice your mind transforming daily, but the effects of the mental exercises are obvious now. You feel strong enough to deal with your DMA situation and overcome any obstacles that seemed impossible before you started these exercises.

The only decision you made was to go walking and then running regularly. You didn't have to decide to change your physique, but it happened anyway.

The only decision you made was to follow these mental exercises. You didn't have to decide to strengthen your mind, but it happened anyway.

Just by running regularly, you transform your body shape, without consciously willing it to happen. Even if you didn't intend it to happen, once you started to run, you could not stop the inevitable transformation in your physical body.

Just by repeating the mental exercises regularly, you transformed your mind, without concentrating on making it happen. Even if you didn't intend it to happen, once you started the mental exercises, you could not stop the inevitable outcome and your mind from getting stronger.

Running transformed your body.
The mental exercises transformed your mind.

By running your physical appearance changed, and your heart and lungs were transformed too.

By doing the mental exercises, your conscious mind changed, and your subconscious mind was transformed too.

₪

When you begin the mental exercises it's unlikely you will notice the difference in your thoughts or emotions on a day-to-day basis. However, as you continue doing them regularly, a day will come, maybe several weeks from now, when you will notice your mind is stronger and you are feeling more positive.

This is inevitable for almost everyone who follows this course, the human mind works the same way for most of us and there are seldom any exceptions.

You may experience days when it feels like you have fallen back into old and more negative thought patterns, but this is perfectly normal and part of the way the mind adjusts to remove these old subconscious ideas for good.

While we are working away to rid ourselves of these outdated beliefs, they can surface at any time. This can be to remind us of the things that don't serve us anymore and to make sure we want to remove them permanently.

If you have an odd bad day, try to remember that your mind is just weeding out the past, and the old outdated ideas that DMA created in your mind.

There will be times when these old ideas try to gain back the control they once had over you, but, when you recognise this, it gives you the chance to reject them again, and possibly for the final time.

The day will come when they are no longer in your subconscious and therefore never able to surface again. After that, the destructive mindset created by DMA, and these old negative ideas will be a thing of the past.

Fleeting ghosts of ideas that you can honestly say have no hold of you anymore.

The idea of surrendering to situations you would have given in to in the past, will just not enter your head. You'll have a new mindset, that will only seek solutions to work toward long-term happiness instead of short-term respite from abuse.

The improvements gained by repeating any exercise are similar, whether it's physical exercise or mental exercise. Your body becomes stronger, as it responds to exercise because it simply has no choice. Your mind becomes stronger, as it responds to mental exercises because it simply has no choice. You cannot fail if you keep doing them ... every day.

We have been taught the benefits of physical exercise, but not the benefits of mental exercise, which is more important to ensure complete well-being, mind and body.

At this point you may be thinking, 'That sounds too easy, too good to be true'. But where do you think a thought like that would come from ... your Inner Abuser?

₪

Using advanced technology available today it is possible to prove that every time you work with these exercises, it can help to rewire the circuits in your brain, constructing pathways for more positive thoughts as it does so. All you have to do is wholeheartedly want the change, then do the exercises regularly. After that, change is inevitable.

Dr Joe Dispenza, is an international scientist, lecturer, researcher, corporate consultant and author. He has been invited to speak in more than thirty-two countries on five continents. He has travelled the globe, using scientific equipment on his students to measure the changes that certain thought processes have on the human brain. He has had the same results all over the world; we are all capable of replacing 'negative' self-beliefs, even those created by mental abuse, with a new more positive mindset. Exercising your mind using repetitive positive mental stimulus is a great way to achieve this. The importance is repeating them regularly, nothing more.

Try not to allow your Inner Abuser to cherry-pick from the exercises while ignoring others. Do them all, in the order they are set out, for the best results.

Don't let your Inner Abuser convince you that you are cured for all time because you feel better over a few days or a few weeks. Remember, this is designed to overcome DMA forever, not to help you feel good temporarily. If DMA has been influencing your thoughts for some time now, it's important to use this book the way it is set out and intended. Don't cut corners, your Inner Abuser will be desperate to convince you to do just that.

The exercises are simple. Used correctly, they work every time.
Medical pills only work if you keep taking them.
These exercises only work if you keep doing them.

The only difficulty you will find is overcoming your Inner Abuser's attempts to stop you from doing them regularly.
Try to make sure you don't let it get in the way.

Regular Repetition.
As simple as that.
Regular Repetition.
No more complicated than that.
Regular Repetition.
It works and it works every time.
Regular Repetition.

That's it.

Your Inner Abuser may jump in here, with reasons and excuses like … 'overcoming something in your mind is all good and well, but you still have to free yourself from your partner physically, find a new place to live and rebuild your life while trying to find enough money to do so'. Ideas like this are the product of a negative mindset. Once that is transformed, you will start to find the belief and new ways to overcome these things.

It has taken a long time for your Inner Abuser to create the way you see the world, but you can start to take back control of your thoughts and feelings from now on.

Repetition is the Key to Success

I am reminded of a woman who was recovering well by using these exercises but allowed her Inner Abuser to regain control and decided to stop doing them. She had managed to remove herself physically from her abuser, bought a new house, and enjoyed the freedom of doing what she wanted when she wanted. She went from a fearful miserable existence to one where she had the opportunity to create a happier life.

However, when she stopped taking the time to do these exercises, she slumped and succumbed to the re-emergence of her Inner Abuser's guilt and doubt. Before she realised it, she was back living with her abusive partner. That same abusive partner, who she said later, increased his ill-treatment from mental abuse to financial abuse, physical abuse and sexual abuse. Her story, and many like it, is the reason this book was created.

- These mental exercises have helped thousands of people around the world to have better, happier lives.
- Your Inner Abuser will attempt to get you to rush things, so be ready to fight that desire.
- Your Inner Abuser might make you feel the book is not working.
- Your Inner Abuser might try to stop you from using this book.
- Remind yourself of this before you start, recognising any negative thoughts your Inner Abuser creates as they appear.
- By following the exercises in this book and using them daily you will soon find it easier to remain in a positive state of mind.

ONE LAST WORD BEFORE YOU BEGIN

Some of us have had longer or more intense conditioning than others, so the recovery time will vary for everyone too. This can also depend on how much you use the exercises each day. The results can still be achieved, but the timescale will vary.

Just as a weak body has little defence from a physical assault, a weak mind has little defence from a mental assault.

Your mind has to be sharp, strong and clear, and these particular exercises have been combined to help you achieve that.

Good food only nourishes the body when you continue to eat it, return to junk food and the body will soon become undernourished and susceptible to ill health and disease.

Failure to continue making these exercises a part of your daily life from now on will allow your mind to become susceptible to thoughts and actions produced by your Inner Abuser.

Good thoughts nourish the mind, bad ones perish it.

Remember the story of the two wolves fighting for control in your head, the one you feed is the one that wins.

To win your battle with the effects of DMA, only feed the white wolf.

Domestic Mental Abuse

CHAPTER 12

THE EXERCISES

CURIOSITY KILLED THE CAT

I know many of you will have skipped ahead to see what these exercises are all about, and I can't blame you. I would be desperate to find a way out of an abusive relationship too. But skipping past all the information you need before being able to use these exercises successfully is not the way to do it.

I'm sorry, but it won't work that way.

Go back, and make your way through the chapters until you reach this point, or you risk losing the ability for this book to help you the way it can. Don't be the cat in that old saying. Go back, and you'll get here soon enough.

Exercise One
DEEP BREATHING

Right about now your Inner Abuser might be saying,

'What?.......... you've managed to make it to this point in the book just to be told to breathe deeply?'

There is more to it than that, these exercises are simple but a lot more powerful than you may realise at first. This is a beauty and a curse. The beauty is, that these exercises are simple and they do work. The curse is, they are so simple, that it's easy for your Inner Abuser to convince you, that they won't work at all!

Try to ignore your Inner Abuser when it appears, because deep breathing is a very important exercise that can help you take control of your thoughts, effectively allowing you to govern what you think about. This is paramount, if you don't take control of your thoughts, your Inner Abuser will and that is what created your present state of mind, and the current situation you find yourself in.

Think about this.

Deep breathing isn't natural if you haven't been exercising vigorously, is it? When was the last time you found yourself deep breathing when you were relaxing? As humans, we have to consciously think about doing it. No other animal can consciously **decide** to do some deep breathing to calm itself at a time of stress or anxiety, but we can. We can **choose** to do it any time we want, and once you realise how beneficial it is, you will want to make it part of your life from now on.

Deep breathing is something we have to make a conscious effort to think about, it doesn't come naturally, we need to become conscious of our thoughts, and decide to do it.

It is a **conscious** decision.

Once we focus on that conscious decision, we have to **choose** to do it, or our body will simply keep on breathing normally. Most of us don't know the full benefits of taking a few minutes several times throughout the day to calm ourselves down, which helps us to look at any situation we find ourselves in, a bit more clearly.

The conscious decision to do some deep breathing is the moment we begin to take control of the troubling thoughts we are having at that time. Being conscious of our breathing brings us back into the present moment and takes our mind away from any negative thoughts of the past, or the future. Deep breathing is a very powerful tool. You cannot fight DMA or your Inner Abuser effectively, without taking control of your thoughts.

I've never met anyone who wants to have thoughts that create fear, anxiety, guilt or shame.

Once we learn to recognise when these destructive thoughts appear, we can **choose** to replace them with positive ones. Practising deep breathing helps to calm us down, distance us from negative thoughts and create space for a more positive frame of mind to emerge.

Remember, the full control of your thoughts has been hijacked by DMA and your Inner Abuser, you have to take this control back if you want to make better decisions from now on.

However, there is more to it.

People always advise others to take a deep breath at a time of stress or anxiety.
This is why.

'Deep breathing calms your mind and relaxes your body' ... exactly what you need when you are scared, stressed, under pressure, or feel you just can't cope.

We have to learn to **remind ourselves** to breathe deeply. It sounds simple but this will not happen automatically, **you** have to make a conscious decision to do it.

If you feel yourself questioning how worthwhile this will be, remember, that your Inner Abuser is never far away in these early days of recovery, and it will try to convince you that anything **designed to help you**, is not going to work **for you**. Stay alert to any negative thoughts or emotions, recognise them and ignore them as you read on. Before you start the exercise be aware of how you are feeling.

Read through all the following directions for the exercise before you begin.

1. If possible sit or lie down, this is important when you first practise this exercise (you may become light-headed with the extra oxygen intake it creates).
2. Close your eyes.
3. During this exercise, breathe in your nose and out of your mouth.
4. Start by taking some breaths that are just slightly deeper than normal.
5. Be aware of the air going in and out and your body relaxing as you do this.
6. **Once you feel slightly more relaxed, breathe smartly in your nose, filling your diaphragm and lungs to a count of four. Then hold it for a count of seven and breathe out (slower) to a count of eight, emptying your lungs completely if possible.**
7. Do this four times and then return to what feels like a natural breath for you.
8. Think about how you feel after completing this exercise, check if your body is slightly more relaxed, then check if your mind feels clearer too.

IMPORTANT NOTE: you may feel light-headed during this exercise, this is caused by the extra oxygen intake going to your brain. (That's why it is best to be sitting or lying down.) As the weeks go by, you will become accustomed to the increase of oxygen while you do this exercise and any light-headed feeling should lessen.

Now think about this.

When you are ill and your doctor gives you a course of antibiotics, do you spend the days constantly asking yourself, 'Do I feel better yet?'

You might get to day two, three or maybe four and there will come a moment when you notice you are beginning to feel the antibiotics working and you are on the road to recovery. It doesn't happen overnight.

So be careful not to keep asking yourself, 'Am I feeling better yet?' every time you do any of these exercises. In the same way, you would follow the antibiotic prescription and take them several times a day, you should also do this exercise several times a day (at least). It takes no time at all and it's not difficult, it is just repetitive. Write down in the space below four times of the day you will do this exercise.

(I will suggest … 'When I wake up', and. .. 'Before I go to sleep'. You decide on 2, 3, 4 and 5)

1. When I wake up.
2.
3.
4.
5.
6. Before I go to sleep.

… you now have a choice of four out of six possible times to do this exercise.

If you are happy to do it more often, that will be even more beneficial but four is a bare minimum. As with all these exercises, the more you do them, the quicker you will feel calmer and more positive throughout the days to follow.

Once you get into a routine, you can do it anywhere, sitting, lying down or even standing up. On the bus or the train, before and after your meals, and any other time you have a few minutes to yourself. If you do this for twenty-one days, it should become a habit. By then you will have added the next exercises to your new routine.

Don't beat yourself up if you forget, just do it as soon as you remember, and eventually, it will become as natural as getting out of bed in the morning.

It is important to become so familiar with the act of deep breathing, you can slip into it naturally.

That's it, exercise one, is simple but more effective than you may realise at the moment, so do not skip over it, all of the exercises are designed to enhance the effect of the others but more importantly, are designed to have a positive effect on your subconscious.

You may think this seems too simple to have any effect on your mood or your life, but remember, DMA negatively alters your subconscious, without you realising it, or noticing any changes happening. The operation to reverse that adverse change works the same way … only in reverse. You won't notice that positive change happening either, but one day, you will wake up and notice a difference in your mindset.

You were not aware of the negative impact DMA was having on your subconscious, and in the same way, you may not be aware of the positive impact these exercises are having either. That is normal, it would be very unusual to feel noticeably better, right away.

You have faith in antibiotics curing you, even though you may not feel any different in the first few days, so try to achieve that same faith in these exercises, whether you feel any different in the early weeks or not. It may not be until you begin to feel mentally stronger, that you realise the power of these exercises to change your life.

Along the way, your Inner Abuser will try to sabotage the process, but this will diminish as you continue to get stronger.

Take a little time to think about this …
I'm sure we would all agree that this first exercise is very simple to do … and very simple to carry out.

If you find you doubt the ability of this exercise to help change your mind, ask yourself, 'Why am I questioning this? It's such a quick exercise, so why am I resisting so much?' The resistance is not from your Authentic Self, it is from your Inner Abuser, and, for the moment, it may still have too big an influence on your mind.

Have you ever asked your doctor, 'How is this box of little pills going to help me feel better?'

No? That's because we have been conditioned to believe a doctor will know what pills to give us and we usually accept their decision without much resistance. This is part of social conditioning, most of us just accept certain aspects of our lives as fact without the least idea *why* we accept them.

Unfortunately, we have not been conditioned to accept that we can reprogramme our own minds, using certain techniques and mental exercises. This is why our Inner Abuser finds it easy to create doubt about the effectiveness of this type of therapy. So if you are feeling resistant or underwhelmed at this first exercise, you're normal! The main thing is, that you brush off the resistance and continue, regardless of the doubt your Inner Abuser might try to create.

Regular deep breathing will calm your brain, relax your body and awaken your conscious mind. The only way to find this out is to make it part of your daily routine.

So, if your Inner Abuser convinced you to skip past it, go back and do this first breathing exercise now.

> *If YOU want to change your life, YOU have to change.*
> *Begin practising Exercise One, throughout the day, every day,*
> *and try not to move on to Exercise Two …*
> *Until you manage a full week of this new breathing regime.*

Repetition of positive mental exercises is the way to beat the effects of DMA properly, but if you try to do too much too quickly, you may not achieve the proper results. Impatience is a friend of the Inner Abuser, not your Authentic Self. You may think you are helping yourself get over DMA quicker by rushing through these exercises and trying to start them all at the same time…. but it simply won't work … slow down and believe in the process if you want to beat DMA properly. You'll soon be glad you did. Introduce and master these exercises one by one, before doing the next one.

Exercise Two

By now you should have been practising Exercise One for at least a week so that it feels familiar, before adding Exercise Two.

After completing Exercise One …

… take a minute to allow your breathing to return to normal.

Regardless of how simple they seem, these exercises are based on the latest neuroscience. They are proven to change the way our minds have been programmed by past events and can create a new positive mindset in the future. They are ideal for anyone who has experienced conditioning through mental abuse.

Let's go

To begin with, do this after Exercise One, just once in the morning and once before going to sleep.

You will need to use a notepad for this. Writing things down has more impact on the mind, and it helps to reprogramme your subconscious. It's the subconscious that runs our day-to-day lives, which is why it is so important to fill it with positive thoughts. By reprogramming the information we store in it, our lives can be based on positive thoughts, not negative ones.

When we wake up in the morning, we don't need to think, 'Okay, now I have to push the duvet off and swing round to put my feet on the ground, then I will need to flex my leg muscles so that I can stand up', we just do it. The subconscious is our personal automatic pilot and it runs our lives a lot more than we realise. These exercises work on our subconscious and therefore influence a large part of our daily lives. They help to create a new database of positive thoughts, emotions and feelings.

If you hear that little voice telling you, 'This will never work for you', ask yourself, 'What is that idea based on? Why is this trying to stop me from giving these mental exercises a chance to work?'

Remember that removing negative thoughts from your mind and stopping them from running your life in the future is the whole reason for doing this course.

₪

Back to the exercise.

When you do this for the first time it doesn't matter what part of the day it is, after that, try to do it first thing in the morning and last thing at night (after your deep breathing).

On your notepad, write down five things you are grateful for over the past twenty-four hours. It can be as simple as a cup of coffee, or a smile from someone you passed in the street, it could be that you feel healthy or that you have discovered this book, or just that you were able to get out of bed this morning.

These are just examples and although you can use them it is important to choose things you are grateful for in your own life and write them down. This might seem more difficult than it sounds at first, that's because it is a new concept compared to the way you have been thinking previously. You may find yourself tripping through your memories of the last twenty-four hours wondering 'What can *I* really be grateful for these days?'. It doesn't matter if it takes some time to complete the first time, that's perfectly normal.

Keep thinking until you come up with five things from the past day that you are grateful for, before moving on.

This will become a lot easier as you repeat the exercise in the days to come, soon you will rattle off ten things without any problem, but for now and possibly the first couple of weeks, just five things will do.

Write them down.

Once you do this, read them out loud, several times, taking time to think about each one before you move on.

Now look at each one in turn and spend a few seconds thinking about how that moment made you feel and the gratitude you have for that particular point in time.

This might not feel very natural to you, in fact, it could feel uncomfortable for the first few days. Try to ignore any feelings of resistance, they are remnants of the old you, the one you are leaving behind, and the one that subconsciously, doesn't believe you deserve happiness.

It may be worth asking yourself this question, 'Why am I finding it difficult to think of things I enjoyed, and relive them in my mind again?'

The answer is this, DMA has conditioned your subconscious to think negatively, so much so that you may almost 'feel guilty' just thinking about positive things.

As you do these exercises, you will find thinking positively no longer feels strange or uncomfortable … It's a process that always works if you keep at it.

Look over your gratitude list and relive each of them for a few moments again now.
When you do this exercise, try to think of different things each time, this will have a better impact on your subconscious. Be genuinely grateful every time you do this exercise. If you cut corners, you will only be cheating yourself. Worse than that, you will dilute your ability

to defeat the effects of DMA. If you have skipped over any part of this exercise, make an effort to go back and focus on your five reasons for gratitude one more time. If it feels difficult, be sure this will get easier in the days to come. The first time you do this exercise will take more effort, although it can depend on what has been going on around you at that time.

Incorporate this exercise into the daily habit you have already established with the first exercise. Do Exercise One (deep breathing) at least four times a day, and add this gratitude exercise twice a day, every morning and evening.

Thinking back, do you remember when you started feeling things were not quite right in your relationship? Could you believe back then, that the person you chose to share your life with would use mental conditioning that could eventually cause you to feel fear, guilt, anxiety, shame, isolation, desperation or despondency in the future? Like many other women, you probably never thought anyone you trusted would try to manipulate your mind in this way.

Just like then, when you look back in the weeks or months to come, you won't remember the exact moment you began to feel better and more positive, you will realise it has happened but you won't be able to say exactly when it happened.

This is how programming or reprogramming the mind works ... we just have to keep doing the exercises and let it happen. And it will.

These exercises are subtly reversing the effects of your partner's abuse and they work within the subconscious. You are rebuilding what has been torn down. Your self-confidence, self-esteem and the belief you have in yourself will return. As you practise each day, even if you don't feel it to begin with, your subconscious is changing.

Simple but powerful.

It is not necessarily how often you do the exercises in one day, as long as you do the minimum required, it is doing them *every single day* that will make the difference. Of course, the more times the better.

Doing them continuously 24/7 for a week may help a little in the short term, but will not help in the long term. You have to do them **consistently**. You don't need to do them more often than recommended, but you have to do them every day **consistently** ... perseverance is the key.

Put these two exercises together and practise them for a week before adding Exercise Three to your new daily routine.

It is important to remind yourself that these exercises will help you more than you might realise at this point, but it is also important that you look forward to doing them, and don't allow your Inner Abuser to label them as a chore ... you have to want this change, or change will not happen. That means you have to tell yourself you want to do these exercises too.

Exercise Three

When you are worried about something it can be very hard not to think of it every moment of the day and this can be quite exhausting.

If you are trying to find a solution to a problem to resolve it, then that is worth spending time contemplating. But, if your mind keeps getting drawn towards something you don't want to happen or something that has already happened and upsets you, then these thoughts are not worthwhile. Once we recognise these destructive thoughts when they appear, we can practice how to stop them and their negative influence on our emotions.

Take this moment to understand what worry really is …
'Thinking about something that you don't want to happen.'
Worry is like a rocking chair, you are moving all day (mentally) but you never get anywhere.
Will worrying change the outcome of the situation at all?
How does worrying make you feel?
Fearful? Anxious? Upset? Scared? Frustrated? Angry?
Do you like feeling any of these emotions?
Do they serve you?

I hope your answer was no. There is absolutely no good reason to worry, but most of us do it far too often. Those of us who have been mentally or emotionally abused do it even more. It clouds our judgements and has an impact on our mental health.
Why on earth would we want to worry about things all the time?
Really. Why do we do it?
I would like you to think about this question, why do we worry?

₪ ₪ ₪

When you see three of these symbols together, you know I want you to think about this question for a while … it's important.

₪

We have been conditioned to worry. It is part of the old redundant 'fight or flight' survival mechanism, it prepares us for the unexpected, but nowadays a 'fight or flight' situation is something we rarely need to consider. However, when we worry, it can create this type of response, releasing hormones designed to help us in dangerous situations but are counterproductive to our mindset, when we are simply sitting in the house … worrying.

Take a moment to think how it would feel if you had nothing in the world to worry about … imagine how it would feel.
What would each day without a worry in the world feel like?

Disregarding your present situation, use your mind to imagine having no worries at all. Try to do this for the next five minutes, before reading on. Think how amazing life would be without a care in the world, this is an important part of these exercises, so don't skip it … immerse yourself in the idea that you have no worries and how that would feel. Do this for five minutes right now … remember haste is a sign the Inner Abuser is influencing you so slow down … then read on …

₪

Think about this … when we worry, we are visualising unwanted future events … then we continuously run them over in our minds. However, most of them never happen. So why do it? Start today and make a decision not to worry about possible events in the future that you have no control over. Things that rarely turn out as bad as your Inner Abuser suggests.

Why not start to visualise good things happening in the future? It's your mind, even if presently you are thinking these good things might not happen, it still feels good to visualise them, doesn't it?

What would you rather think about …
 … something that makes you concerned or frightened and you have no control over …
 … or something that makes you feel relaxed and joyful?

You may not have realised it, but this is a choice your mind is making subconsciously because you are not becoming conscious enough to tell yourself, 'Stop this, it is not serving me and it is not helping me, stop it now'. It **IS** your choice. Remember the chapter heading, 'Who Chooses Your Thoughts'?

How amazing would it be if your mind could take a short holiday from all its worries? This is why I asked you to imagine what it would feel like to have no worries.
 Simply not think about them at all … or better still, how good would it be to get rid of them permanently? Really, how would that feel?

We have been conditioned to worry throughout our lives. Much of the news on the TV, radio, internet and in the papers is 'bad news'. This conditions us to think more bad things than good happen in the world. When we watch or listen to the news, we are being directed to things that happened on the other side of the world. Things that will not influence our own lives but sometimes we become concerned about these far-off events.

We are then worrying about something we have no control over, we cannot change and that will probably have no impact on **our** lives.

When we do this we are having negative thoughts for no reason. We are being subconsciously conditioned to think about things that will never affect us and we have no control over. When we realise this, we can become more selective about where we place our attention.

DMA works the same way. A partner repeating how useless, ugly, pathetic, annoying or stupid you are, eventually creates an uneasy demoralised feeling that stays in our subconscious. (Have you ever noticed that the news repeats itself over and over again throughout the day? It's called conditioning.) Your partner might believe all the nasty things he says to you, but you don't need to believe them. However, when he repeats it often enough your subconscious starts to accept it unless you consciously take control of your thoughts. When DMA undermines your reality, you start to worry about him, the things he says, and the things he does.

When you are worried about him all the time, you are no longer concerning yourself with what is best for **you** and that is exactly what he wants.

The way your DMA partner has conditioned you to see the world has to be reversed. That includes worrying about things you have no control over. It's time to stop worrying and take control of your mind.

You can teach yourself to do this by staying more conscious, and choosing what you think about.

You can condition yourself to recognise and reject 'worries' as a useless and negative form of thinking. By rejecting these thoughts as you become aware of them, you will diminish their influence on your mind and give it a well-earned rest.

Exercise Three is simply to encourage you to watch your thoughts, and if they are not serving you, choose to think about something else, something that makes you happy, or something from the gratitude list you make each morning.

When you recognise a negative thought, say to yourself, 'I don't need to think about that just now, it isn't serving me.'

₪

This exercise is not something you do for five or ten minutes twice a day, it is constant, staying alert to unhelpful thoughts that seem to appear from nowhere, and fend them off. You will benefit tenfold from the effort you put in to repel thoughts that don't serve you. Put Exercise Three in motion as you go through your day from now on. As you persist with watching your thoughts, you will find you begin to worry less. This is over a period of time, but it does happen. So persevere.

Exercise Four

*'I can't stop thinking about it!' ... But how hard have you tried to stop?
To become good at something, you need to practise ... a lot.*

This is two exercises, one you have to develop, and one you can use when you feel like it.

Many of the negative thoughts that run through our heads on a daily basis, are unhelpful, even damaging to our mental well-being.

Even when we recognise these negative thoughts it is still difficult to completely stop them for more than a few seconds. This is an exercise where all you do is 'watch' your thoughts and they melt away themselves.

When you recognise you are having disturbing thoughts (and worries), the first thing to do is the deep breathing from Exercise One ... this will calm your mind, lower your heart rate and blood pressure.

Part 1

This will test your imagination, and focus your mind. You may recognise it.

Become aware of your conscious thoughts. Imagine you are a miniature-sized observer, sitting on a stage at the back of your head, looking towards a screen on the inside of your forehead. This screen is where the show is. The show is your thoughts as they appear and disappear on the screen, but you are merely observing them, you are not your thoughts. You are separate and you are observing them in turn as they appear.

You are not judging them, not liking or disliking them, just watching them go by. Not trying to change them, or replace them, just watching them. Not feeling them, just watching the thoughts as they come and go on the screen. Don't attach any feeling or emotion to them just simply observe them.

You will need to get used to this idea before you can do it properly, unless you have been practising since you read about it in the earlier chapter. It does take a bit of practice, but once it's mastered, it can be a game-changer. Soon, it will be easy to feel yourself on that tiny stage, watching the thoughts on a screen, but not being part of them. Just as you would watch a film but are not one of the characters, you are just watching them, not judging them, just watching them pass. Not feeling them, just watching them pass.

They are not you, they are thoughts generated by a part of your mind that is difficult to access at the moment, but they are just thoughts and can only hold the power you allow them to have.

As you watch, you may find they slow down, and may even stop appearing altogether. If this happens, carry on watching, ready to observe any more thoughts that are generated and arrive on the screen. All this time you must remain conscious of being the one on the stage, separate from the thoughts on the screen but just watching them. It may not be easy to keep your concentration, but as you practise, it will become effortless. When you notice your focus has wandered, just bring it back to the words as they appear on the screen.

It is quite demanding to stay focused on this exercise, but making space in our head where we simply watch the thoughts our mind creates without being part of them, forms a new structure to the way our brain operates.

This is quite tricky, to begin with.

You might want to replace the image on the stage with a younger, carefree version of yourself. Whatever image you use, become it, sitting on the stage and simply watching the thoughts go by.

Begin to immerse yourself in these exercises, practising daily. As you do, your subconscious mind has no option but to change the way it operates.

Separating yourself from your thoughts helps you to understand many thoughts are generated randomly in our subconscious and a lot of them are ones we don't want.

Using this exercise stops us from getting involved with the constant mental chatter our mind engages in throughout the day. Mastering this helps quieten the mind and brings us back to the present moment. As you use it, you will begin to understand that many of the thoughts you have from moment to moment are unnecessary. Forced on you by a subconscious mind that will not stop generating unhelpful ideas every minute of every day … until you train it to slow down and stop, every now and then.

Focus, repetition and consistency are the keys to reprogramme a new way of thinking.

Part 2
Visualisation to Stop Your Partner from Dominating Your Thoughts

Close your eyes. Imagine you are sitting in a comfortable armchair and your abusive partner (or ex), is standing right in front of you, imagine them life-size and in full colour. Look them up and down, and observe their face and the clothes they have on. After around 30 seconds, or when it feels right, imagine the colour fades out of them until they are standing there in shades of grey, like a black and white photograph.
Now imagine them further away from you, and now the size of a child. Take up to 30 seconds to visualise this, don't rush it, they are now a small distant grey figure in your mind.

Now, imagine they have moved even further away … right to the horizon, very small and very far away, a tiny dot on the horizon.

Now, watch that tiny image disappear over the horizon, and they are gone.

(Adapted from the book *'How to Mend Your Broken Heart'* by Paul McKenna and Hugh Willbourn.)

Repeating this, as often as you need to, will help you stop thinking about your ex whenever he keeps reappearing in your mind. To begin with, you may only get respite for thirty seconds, or a minute, or two. Don't get upset at this, just do the whole thing again as soon as you become aware that he has returned to your thoughts.

You may need to do this a lot, to begin with, but do not get frustrated. How far do you think you would get if I asked you to take a ride on a unicycle for the first time?

Practice.

Imagining your first attempt at riding a unicycle might help you understand we may have to practise some things more than others to master them. This applies as much to our mind as to our body.

Think of your mind as a unicycle, and try not to expect too much on your first 'ride'. Everything comes with practice.

This means there may be a lot of repetition, to begin with, and until you are more in control of your thoughts. Once you get good at these exercises, it will only require routine revision, to stay in control.

The more you watch your thoughts, the better use you can make of your mind and your time.

Every time you practise these exercises, you are rewiring your subconscious, making it easier to focus on the positive aspects of your life without any effort.

As you continue using the exercises, this will happen automatically. One day, you will feel there has been a shift in your mindset. You will start to believe in yourself and what you are capable of. You may feel you are at the very beginning of this journey, but if you have been practising these exercises regularly, there will already be a shift in your mindset, even if you are not aware of it yet.

Now, you are heading in the right direction, instead of the wrong one.

Try to take these exercises on board and consistently implement them from now on. Don't move on to Exercise Five for at least a week after adding these new recommendations to your routine. If you read on now, all you are doing is reading, you are not learning, practising or changing. Reading will not change a thing in your life. Practising the mental exercises will. Think about this before you continue to read.

Exercise Five

DMA works by repetition, if your partner tells you that you're ugly, stupid or useless enough times, your subconscious starts to believe it. If he is not as blunt as that but says things like, 'Go and put a bit of makeup on for goodness sake', or, 'Do I have to explain everything to you?', or, 'Can't you do anything right?', it will still affect you. An abuser's use of words can be subtle as well as direct, but they all harm the subconscious.

Your subconscious eventually surrenders to the repetition of the words and phrases he uses and somewhere in the depths of your mind, you begin to believe his rhetoric.

Just as you can't remember when his insults began to affect you, you might not notice your mind beginning to shift in the opposite direction as you practise these exercises.

Do you ever notice the exact moment you fall asleep? No! But the fact is, you end up being asleep. That is how subtly the mind works sometimes.

₪

If you are wondering when you will see a difference, it's worth remembering the woman who was finding it so difficult to stop herself from returning to her ultra-abusive partner.

When I went to see her, she was curled up in the corner of the room, in her pyjamas, her face stained with tears from hours of crying, saying she couldn't cope with … 'all the stuff going on because I left him'.

I asked her to give me half an hour of her time and to do exactly what I asked … she agreed to pull herself together and try to follow my instructions …

… the next day she sent me a picture, looking radiant and well, with the caption, 'I feel transformed, I'm off to see some girlfriends for lunch, thank you so much.'

That half-hour I asked her for was spent repeating this exercise …

I went over it first and asked the woman to copy me, repeating the words out loud without concentrating on their meaning. Just repeat what she heard me say out loud.

It's easy to underestimate the ability of these exercises to transform your mind. I am about to ask you to do a simple thing right now, however, you may find you have a major rush of resistance to it. The level of this resistance can be an indication of how much you have to overcome in your subconscious.

To rid yourself of the changes DMA caused, this type of resistance has to be cleared.

₪

Don't worry if you can't bring yourself to believe these words, most people that do this exercise for the first time tell me it feels very awkward to say these words out loud.

Take your time to do this exactly as it is explained, the benefits are not easy to comprehend but they may change your life just like the woman mentioned above. Don't get into a big debate in your head about this, just repeat the words without attaching your thoughts to them …

1. Find a big mirror, (in the future have one prepared beside you), if you want to do this exercise any time during the day, be sure to carry a small mirror with you.
2. Sit down in front of the large mirror and get comfortable, take a few deep breaths … and then …
3. Look into your own eyes in the mirror, and take your time to study the true colour of them.
4. Look into your pupils, look beyond the surface, and deep into your eyes. Your Authentic Self is centred deep inside. Your true self-belief is there.
5. Don't think about the next words or their meaning, keep staring into the reflection of your own eyes and just say out loud … **I like you.**
6. Now keep looking into your eyes and say out loud … **I really like you.**
7. Then say out loud … ***your first name e.g. Carol*, I really like you.**
8. Do this without thinking about the words or what they mean, just do it now, and repeat all three parts, twice more.
9. Continue to say the words again but still do not think about their meaning. Now do this slowly, ten times.
10. After you have repeated these phrases ten times, think about this; it has probably taken no more than a couple of minutes to do this exercise. (If it felt like a very uncomfortable couple of minutes, you are not alone. This is because you're not used to communicating with yourself in this way. This awkward feeling will soon fade as you go on.)

11. Don't let the meaning of the words put you off, no matter how they make you feel, find a way to say them. Look into your own eyes in the mirror and say it another ten times right now ...

I like you.
I really like you.
(Your name) I really like you.

The important part here is for your ears to hear your voice saying these words. If it feels easier not attaching any further importance to it than that, good. Just get the words out and you will make that important difference to your subconscious.

Any resistance you feel will come from your Inner Abuser. When working to reverse the effects of DMA, the Inner Abuser is never far away, especially in the early stages of recovery. It creates reasons why you should not like yourself, but don't get too distracted, you will soon change that by practising the exercise.

Even if it doesn't feel like it right now, repeating this exercise helps you take control of the conscious and the subconscious, and doing this on a daily basis will change your mindset more than you can believe at this time.

Other people can encourage and support you but no one else can do this for you ... If you find this exercise awkward, it is because you need it more, not less.

The effects mental abuse has on the mind can only be reversed by working within the mind that has been affected. No one else can do this for you and that is why working with these exercises is so important. It's a process that relies on repetition if you want to get results.

If you feel some strange urge to bypass this mirror work, it is a direct reflection of how much this can help you. This exercise can rapidly reprogramme the mind over a short time, but you need to continue working with it for long-term change.

₪

If you carried on reading and didn't try to do this exercise, it is completely understandable, it's not an easy thing for most of us to do, especially women affected by DMA. Even if you find yourself laughing at how ridiculous you might feel or crying as you release some long trapped emotions you just have to get through it, before moving on.

₪

This exercise only takes a few minutes, so try to find time out to do it throughout your day. Above all other exercises, mirror work, if done correctly, can change your mindset as soon as you do it. Sometimes it will take a bit more time to feel the positive effects of it, and if that's the case, just keep looking into the mirror, say the words and put a bit more belief into them each time … you *do* like yourself … so let yourself know it.

I remember the first time I was given morphine after dislocating my shoulder. The pain in my shoulder was excruciating but I was amazed when the injection took the pain away instantly, allowing me to feel relaxed and comfortable. Until then I would never have guessed the incredible difference morphine could have in just a few seconds.

Like morphine, these exercises can have a surprising and quick effect on you too, an effect you cannot guess until you practise them for yourself.

I probably wouldn't have believed anyone that told me morphine could take away that pain in such a remarkable way. Similarly, I have experienced people who could not quite believe this exercise would have such an effect on their self-esteem until they started using it.

It's time to pause and perfect all of the exercises you have learned so far. Revise and use them together for at least a week before moving on. Don't allow your Inner Abuser to ignore this rule. It will be counterproductive.

Your mind can only progress so much over a short period so don't be impatient. This is a process that cannot be rushed. You will find this process works a lot better and creates a more permanent change if you allow these exercises time to sink in before moving on from here.

Consistency and Repetition

₪

Exercise Six

You will affect the ability of the book to help you if you read on, without repeating the exercises you have learned so far for at least a week.

This will feel very familiar to you, however, you may find a higher resistance to it than you expect, even though Exercise Six is just Exercise Five with a single word changed.

As before, try not to think about the meaning of the words, just say them out loud and do the exercise.

1. Sit in front of the mirror as before, take a few deep breaths, take time to look deep into the reflection of your eyes and say out loud …

I love you.
I really love you
(Your name) I really love you

If you resist, you are most likely concentrating on the meaning of the words, stop this and just say them out loud again …

… and again … up to ten times, but keep looking into the reflection of your eyes the whole time.

Now keep doing it, but this time start to allow yourself to feel the words, try not to think whether it is right or wrong, true or false, don't judge, just feel them as you hear yourself saying them out loud. Feel it, don't judge it.

Observe how hearing the words makes you feel and remember it is always okay for you to hear these words. It is not a crime.

If you do feel it's wrong to say, 'I love you' to yourself, ask yourself why it is wrong?

It is one of the most beautiful things to say to someone else, so why not yourself? Even if it doesn't feel comfortable, find a way to get the words out, and always say them out loud.

Every time you do this it will feel more natural. It's a case of your ears hearing your voice saying the words, and looking into your eyes in the mirror. It is these factors that will make a difference to your subconscious.

You have to use a mirror.

You have to say it out loud.

When you get used to this exercise, start feeling the love you are sending yourself.

It might take you out of your comfort zone, and it may feel like you're faking it, to begin with. Try to get over this by reminding yourself, that your 'comfort zone' is actually just anything you're used to, and not necessarily a comfort at all.

Many women who have been mentally abused are unable to progress in a relationship if their new partner is respectful or considerate towards them. They are so indoctrinated that when they're treated with respect something feels 'wrong'. They are just not used to it. DMA can manipulate a woman's thoughts to such a degree that being treated with consideration can make her feel uncomfortable. Some women overreact to the absence of abuse so much that they can become emotionally abusive themselves. This is their subconscious repeating learned behaviour. It may be that they feel uncomfortable because they don't understand or recognise their new partner's considerate behaviour. It makes them feel uncomfortable.

Being nice to yourself, by telling your reflection, 'I love you' can invoke the same response of rejection or discomfort. The need to reject compliments either from others or your reflection in the mirror will diminish the more you do this exercise.

Make a note that *you* could re-enact behaviour learned from your abuser. In doing so, you may turn away good people, by simply not paying attention to your own words and actions toward them. Do you want to take on the personality of an abuser yourself? Be watchful, and underline this paragraph as a reminder.

₪

You are now a few weeks into the exercises, so let's recap here.

If you managed to ignore the Inner Abuser's attempt to sabotage this new routine, you should feel a little more optimistic about your future. By now you may be able to cope with your present situation better too.

There is still a bit to go, by continuing to repeat the exercises every day, you will develop a stronger mind, more capable of dealing with life's challenges.

Some may not feel all that different in the first few weeks, but there will already be changes in your subconscious mind.

If you started going to the gym three weeks ago, you wouldn't see much difference in your body just yet. That doesn't mean changes haven't happened. The same applies to exercising your mind. Be patient, changes will happen … if … you follow the exercises as directed.

It is so important to make sure you don't slip, take less time over them, or become less focused as you continue the daily routine you have created. Remember, we are working to alter a state of mind that has been conditioned over a long period. Your Inner Abuser will remain in the background, trying to convince you this book is not helping you. As long as you realise this will not happen overnight. Stick to the routine and changes will become evident soon enough.

You should soon be feeling more positive about your future in weeks four to six of this course.

Something to look out for … IMPATIENCE
(another trick of the Inner Abuser)

This is one of the big dangers when dealing with the effects of DMA.

Be careful of impatience. It is always better to do nothing than to do the wrong thing. Your DMA partner will try to use urgency against you if you let him. Watch out for any impatience in your life, either from you or aimed at you. Take a moment to let this sink in, it is important and often overlooked by women who have suffered from DMA.

> Don't let impatience undo your good work.
> Patience is a virtue, a valuable one.

Be careful, your future self might regret any hasty decisions you make now, due to impatience. There is an old saying, 'If in doubt, do nothing.'

If you feel under pressure through impatience, use Exercise One, deep breathing settles the mind and the body. Don't rush it, allow the breathing time to work, it only takes a few moments, but will relax you and bring clarity to a situation. Think about decisions you made in the heat of the moment, that caused more harm than good in the long run. Remind yourself not to have the same kind of knee-jerk reaction again. Recognising bad decisions made because of impatience can prevent you from doing the same again.

If you are unsure of a decision you need to make, give yourself twenty-four hours before returning to it. In that twenty-four hours, use the exercises you have learned so far and don't do anything one way or the other until a full day has passed.

Towards the end of the day, after deep breathing, working with your gratitudes and your mirror work, take a little time to do this …

Exercise Seven

Imagine you have a big choice to make and you rush the decision on it. Now imagine your future self, a week later.

- Take time to visualise this, how are you feeling a week from now?
- Is your future self still happy you made that decision?
- Did that decision benefit you at the time you made it?
- Is it still benefiting you a week later?
- What happened in that week, as a result of making that decision?
- Is your future self still happy you made that decision?

₪

Now, take the time to imagine your future self a month later.

- Is your future self happy about what has happened in that month?
- Take time to visualise what the consequences of that decision have been.
- Do you wish you had taken the time and made a different decision?

₪

Imagine your future self, six months after making that decision.

- How would your future self be feeling?
- What happened in the six months after making that decision?
- Is your future self happy you made that decision?
- Take time to visualise what the consequences of that decision may have been.
- How do you feel about making that decision now?

So by then, has it worked out well or was it a bad decision?

Lastly, have you been truthful to yourself, as time goes by, is your future self going to be happy as a result of that decision?

₪

Now, think about your past, how far back can you remember in your DMA relationship?

This is not about regretting decisions made in the past, it is about making better ones in the future. The fact you now recognise bad decisions in the past means you can make better ones in the future. That is the only reason we are looking back, to learn from those actions, not to dwell on them. The past is gone, we cannot change it and regret is not something that serves us, try not to regret it, try to learn from the past.

If you learn from it, then it will help you make better decisions from now on.

Do you remember key decisions you made a week ago, a month ago, six months ago, a year or even five years ago (if the relationship is that old)?

- Did you decide to stay with him without thinking about the long-term consequences?
- Did you make a decision quickly because you felt you had to?
- Did you take the time back then, to think about how a decision would impact your life now?
- Would you have made different decisions if you could see your situation today?

Bad decisions in the past are okay. You didn't know about the Inner Abuser back then. You may not have known about DMA, or how it affected your mind. And you wouldn't have known how to watch the decisions you were making back then either.

You are not to blame for decisions you made in the past, no one should be held accountable for decisions made under the duress of DMA. **You are blameless.**

That was all before you discovered how DMA can affect your mind, how you think and what you think. It was before you discovered how to reverse the harm DMA causes. **Keep reminding yourself, that you are not responsible** for past decisions and the consequences are not your fault either … few people recognise the stealthy tactics employed by a narcissist early in a relationship. It can take a long time to become aware there is something wrong in your life. You are no different from millions of others who have been deceived in this way. The good thing is, that this book has a system to overcome DMA and all its hidden effects. By just reading this book, you are showing a willingness to change your present situation.

Mark these pages with your pen and return to them whenever you feel you are being forced into a decision by anyone. Take twenty-four hours to think about the situation and until then try not to discuss the subject further.

If in Doubt, do Nothing

Think of Exercise 7 as a lesson in choosing to do nothing. If you do nothing, by default you can't do something you will regret. If you ensure you are not acting under the influence of your Inner Abuser, your decision after twenty-four hours is more likely to be one your future self will be grateful for, not regret you made.

Where DMA is concerned it's better to hold off when you feel anxiety pushing you to make a decision ... try to get used to doing your deep breathing if you feel like this.

Practise the art of saying no or no thanks.

Saying 'no' can empower you and assert yourself to those around you. You can disagree with someone if they are trying to manipulate you. If you feel intimidated by the idea of saying no, begin by refusing less important issues that will not provoke too much of a response.
Say it in a polite but forceful manner. 'No thanks'.

Work up to saying no to more important decisions. Once you commit to saying 'no' in a situation, be careful not to allow that decision to be undermined. As time goes by, saying 'no' will feel more natural and empowering, as you make decisions based on what is best for you, not anyone else.

You may gain some respect when others realise they are not able to manipulate your decision-making.

It's Okay to Say 'No' to Other People Too

It's equally okay to say 'no' to other people who are trying to manipulate you as well. When you are affected by DMA you may find yourself trying to please everyone around you, not just your abusive partner.

A woman who had already left her abusive partner once said to me, 'I know I should make sure I am not emotionally abused by my ex, but I think it's okay to be controlled by my children, isn't it?'

This woman eventually returned to her husband after she became complacent and stopped using the exercises in this book (she said, they had helped her so much she didn't need to keep doing them, which proved not to be the case).

It is worth noting that the three 'children' she thought it was okay to be controlled by were between the ages of 20 and 30 years old. The DMA she had suffered, created the illusion that it was 'acceptable' for certain others to try to control her … but control is just abuse, whoever it's from.

It wasn't obvious to her, that no one, regardless of their connection to you, should be allowed to control or manipulate you. The sad part was, that her partner was not the father of her children, but he had been around long enough for the kids to learn from him and could mimic all his techniques to control their mother's mind. They didn't necessarily recognise they were doing anything wrong especially when their mother capitulated to them almost as much as she did to her abusive partner.

Allowing her children to control (abuse) her was another sign she still had some way to go to overcome the influence DMA still had on her thought process. Even though she had left her abusive partner behind at that time.

Of course, many mothers want to be their children's 'friend', but if she becomes a 'friend' that believes it is okay to allow *them* to be in control, there is still work needed to overcome her Inner Abuser.

In normal circumstances as an adult, it's not usually acceptable for ANY human being to try to control you. These exercises can help you deal with mental abuse from anyone, not just your partner.

Mental abuse, regardless of how subtle, can come from your children, whatever their age. They might not realise what they are doing, but that doesn't mean it's okay for them to do it.

Usually, they are just copying your partner, and don't realise what they are doing. Monkey see, monkey do. By standing strong, acting firm but fair, you are safeguarding yourself from any further abuse and teaching by example. Demonstrating you are no longer willing to stand for any further unreasonable demands from your kids, will show you are no longer willing to be manipulated or controlled.

If your children have witnessed your partner emotionally, verbally, financially or sexually abusing you, they may think these actions are 'normal'. They could also mimic them by directing similar abuse at you or other people, without realising what they're doing. This is a learned behaviour.

Your kids may not have an abusive personality in their genes, but they could end up re-enacting what they witness at a young age. Subconsciously thinking it's acceptable in a relationship when they become adults themselves.

I was affected by this situation as a child. I didn't understand the psychological impact on me until I began researching DMA later in life. DMA has a ripple effect on others in the family, not just the one directly in the firing line.

When you and your children escape your abusive partner, all of you are saved from further psychological conditioning, harrowing home life and the upset he could cause them.

Learn to say 'no'.

Be mindful of your right to say 'no' to *anyone* that tries to impose their will, or places unreasonable demands on you.

EXERCISE 8
Recognising Unhelpful Thoughts and How to Change Them

Why is this important?

If you have been affected by DMA, it is easy to fall back into old ways if you don't continue to work closely with this book. Remember, mulling over old memories or fretting about the future doesn't serve any positive purpose. Allowing your mind to graze through negative aspects of your life will only act against a quick recovery from DMA. You may not have practised diverting your mind away from unpleasant thoughts in the past, but it is a most worthwhile practice, and this will help you do that.

This is a gentle reminder

It is sometimes difficult to keep reminding ourselves about something unseen by the naked eye. Out of sight, out of mind. When we get a bruise or a cut, or even a broken bone, we have the visible presence of the need to treat that part of our body with care and tenderness. But when our minds are affected and in need of TLC, we have no visible reminder that we need to care for them too. It is easy to forget, that where DMA is concerned, above all else, it is the mind we need to handle with care.

The effects of DMA are invisible, but they exist and hamper our ability to return to a normal life even if we escape an abusive partner in the physical sense.

Why would anyone want to keep having thoughts that upset them?

The answer to that is obvious, they wouldn't. We were never taught to observe how our thoughts are making us feel. If we learn to become conscious of our thoughts, we can stop any that are hampering our ability to feel at our best. With some practice we are able to choose what is in our conscious mind but most of us just don't realise it. This allows the thoughts that bring us down to linger in our minds and affect our moods. This is not good for our long-term well-being.

These thoughts are not lingering in our minds because we want to feel bad, they are there because we don't consciously make an effort to address the problem.

It's important to learn how to become the master of our thoughts and therefore our minds.

You may have heard of the word 'mindfulness', in simple terms, it just means being aware of our own minds, and observing our thoughts. Although it is similar to the exercise where we watch our thoughts as they roll across the screen in our heads, this goes a little further …

At several times throughout the day, whenever you remember, ask yourself,

'Are the thoughts I am having right now, making me feel good, or bad?'

Like the other exercises, this will take practice before it becomes a natural part of your day. Many of these exercises seem simple until you realise how much you have to practise to master them. The change they will make to your outlook on life and your ability to make better decisions in the future will be very worthwhile.

Each thought, even though you are not aware of it, affects your subconscious. It doesn't matter if it's one fleeting thought, or a train of them that occupy your mind for hours, they can all still have a lasting impression on your inner mind. Sometimes you can't seem to help returning to a particular theme for days on end, even if it's getting you down.

Negative thoughts store away negative ideas that your Inner Abuser could use against you at a later date, and we can all do with less of them in our minds.

The more you ask yourself how a thought is making you feel, the more you become aware of the ones triggering certain 'feelings'. Feelings are an important indicator of how your mind is working, consciously or subconsciously.

To eliminate bad feelings being created, we have to eliminate the thoughts that cause them. Sounds simple, but we know by now we need to work at these things.

Who would want to be *thinking about* anything that makes them feel bad?

Once we become conscious of negative random thoughts manifesting in our minds, we can practise changing them and choosing what we are going to think about instead.

₪

'It's not that easy', you may say, 'my abusive partner keeps coming into my thoughts and scaring me, even when I don't want to be thinking about him.'

It's okay to feel like that at first, what we are doing right now, is making ourselves aware of our thoughts and how they are making us feel at any given moment in time.

₪

This exercise will help us to recognise these moments and train our minds to think more positively.

- First, write down a list of things that make you feel good and you enjoy.
- Then choose one of them at random.
- Then focus on it, visualise it and expand on it, really immerse yourself in the picture.

Your list can include:
- Places or people, in the present, past or future …
- … or it could be the words of a song you like (singing in your head, or out loud, means you cannot concentrate on other thoughts that may make you feel bad).
- It could be a holiday to a place you've always wanted to go …
- … or a time in the future you can visualise when everything is going well for you.

Using your imagination to create positive thoughts releases endorphins in your body that gives you the 'feel-good factor'. Your body produces endorphins as you immerse yourself in pleasant visualisation.

So it can be a good memory, but it is better to create a scenario for the future, something you have already planned or something you would like to happen. Remember how good your imagination was when you were a child? Well deep down, you still have it, all you need to do is practise using it again. Permit yourself to do this now. Take your time and see what good thoughts you are inspired to have.

₪

I first used this exercise to get myself to sleep when I was going through a difficult situation in my life and disturbing thoughts were constantly keeping me awake.

- Practise watching your thoughts as you go through the day.
- Become aware of your thoughts.
- Are they making you feel bad?
- If so, tell yourself, 'I do not want to feel bad, I am going to stop thinking about this right now'.
- Imagine physically throwing the negative thoughts out of your head.
- Choose something that makes you feel good from your written list.
- Elaborate on the picture you are painting in your mind and immerse yourself in it.

You may get distracted from this new thought quite quickly at first, and find your mind returning to the previous negative thought. That is perfectly normal. Remind yourself that no matter how often this happens you are in control, and you still have the ability to recognise it, stop it and replace it with a good thought from your list.

Practise this exercise any time you are being affected by a negative mindset. This stops any chance of getting caught in a downward spiral or a chain of destructive thinking, which is always a danger to anyone dealing with DMA.

Who chooses your thoughts? … You do, either consciously or subconsciously, so endeavour to master them.

Practice and Repetition

It won't create the perfect headspace overnight, these things take time, but you can look forward to going through a whole day, without your mind creating unhelpful or disturbing thoughts plucked from your subconscious. That day will come if you keep practising this exercise.

Substituting the 'Now Moment' Instead of Visualisation

If you find visualisation difficult, when you realise your thoughts are making you feel bad, you can ask yourself, 'What can I do this very moment to make me feel better?'

Play music, call a friend for a chat, have something healthy you like to eat or take the dog for a walk. Immerse yourself in the present moment, the 'now' moment. Observe your surroundings, and be conscious of what you see, the colours and shapes, the smells or even the feel of whatever comes to hand. Immersing yourself in the 'now' is a very powerful way to clear your mind of all other thoughts, as before, it takes practice to perfect this exercise.

Exercise Nine

Give yourself plenty of time to understand and practise this exercise, it is definitely not something you can read over at speed. Plan to have an hour free before you go any further. It is also best to minimise any form of distraction, put your phone on silent if you can.

To get the desired results, you need time to concentrate on your thoughts and the words you are going to say out loud. Don't go any further if you do not have the free time right now. If you only have a few minutes free just now, practise some of the exercises you have learned already. There is no use rushing through this one, you will not get any benefit if you don't have enough time to understand it or practise it properly.

₪

This exercise is based on EFT, 'Emotional Freedom Technique', and is commonly referred to as Tapping

If you have not heard of EFT previously, the concept may seem a little strange, but that is simply because it is a different approach to improving our mental health. It has no known side effects, unlike many forms of medication.

Try to have an open mind, and again, if you feel doubts about the power of this exercise to reduce the effects of DMA, remind yourself of your Inner Abuser, it's never far away and always trying to sabotage your recovery.

Remember, the subconscious runs our daily lives most of the time.

DMA causes stress, and stress can cause:
- Anxiety
- Depression
- Lack of motivation
- Weight gain
- Weight loss
- Chronic pain
- Digestion system disorders
- Sleeping problems

Using EFT has helped thousands of people tackle all of these issues and can help anyone suffering from the problems in this list caused by DMA. Although it will take a little time to learn this, it only takes a few minutes to do, once you master it.

According to 'The Tapping Solution' website (www.thetappingsolution.com):

> 'After 260,000 plays of our "Releasing Anxiety" tapping meditation video, the average reported reduction of anxiety was 41% in just 9 minutes'

It's great for overcoming stress and anxiety in general, and therefore it's ideal to tackle the negative effects of DMA too.

Tapping is based on modern psychology and ancient Chinese acupressure. First, you focus your thoughts on a negative emotion that's bothering you, it could be anything; fear, isolation, guilt, shame, a bad memory or another unresolved issue you have. Then, while holding this issue in your mind, with your fingertips, you tap on meridian points of the nervous system on your body. Doing this sends a calming signal to your brain, addressing the negative effects of the particular issue you are working on and this relaxes you.

This technique is now regularly used by people around the world to overcome issues they have been troubled with for years and is a great tool to quickly reduce the negative emotions triggered by DMA.

'The Tapping Solution' goes on to say:

'Research is Showing That Tapping Changes D.N.A. Expression, Hormone Production (Particularly Cortisol) and Brain Activation'

It's effective in reducing anxiety and can bring instant relief when mental challenges become overwhelming. It is also an authorised treatment for war veterans suffering from PTSD (post-traumatic stress disorder).

The best way to learn the Tapping technique to perfection is to watch a free video on the internet, there are many and they all show the same procedures. If you can, watch a few before you begin practising it for yourself. Here is a written explanation of how to do Tapping properly.

₪

The Tapping Exercise

You have to address each negative emotion or belief you have, separately. So, if you feel you're not good enough to cope on your own, then address this as one issue. (DMA undermines anyone's ability to believe in themselves).

If you feel guilty (maybe about questioning your partner's use of DMA), address this as one issue. Guilt, created by his DMA, can be a very toxic and debilitating emotion. (It can still be just a series of conditioned thoughts, as a result of mental abuse).

If you feel ashamed about allowing yourself to be manipulated by your partner, you are not alone. However, there are millions of women in DMA relationships; do you think any of those women would have chosen their partner if they were aware of his abusive personality? We can all get deceived by other people's manipulative words and actions.

- If you feel fearful of your abusive partner, or find yourself walking on eggshells (this is usually a result of DMA conditioning).
- If you feel isolated (another result of mind conditioning).
- If you feel helpless (this is a symptom of DMA conditioning).

These are a few of the issues women living with a DMA partner can face, however, if you identify other feelings or beliefs that are causing you to feel negative about your present situation in life, you can address each one, in turn, using EFT.

What are your feelings about your life at present? What are the reasons behind those feelings? Guilt, shame, isolation, fear or something else?

EFT Tapping can be divided into five steps. If you have more than one issue or fear, you can repeat this sequence to address each one in turn and reduce or eliminate the intensity of that negative belief.

As you come up with each issue, write them down, even use the margin of this book to do this, as long as you have them in front of you, it means you don't need to continue to identify them each time you work through them in turn.

Focusing on only one problem at a time, and follow these steps …

1. Choose one of your issues to work on, and decide how intensely you are feeling it is a problem.
On a scale of 0 to 10 (10 being the worst), how much is it bothering you? This scale tells you the level of emotional or even physical pain you feel because of this issue.

By doing this test before the Tapping exercise, you can compare how you feel after it. If the anxiety level was 10, to begin with, and you find it's at 6 after the exercise, you can monitor how much the Tapping has improved your feelings about this issue.

2. Before Tapping, you need to create a phrase that describes what you're trying to overcome.
The phrase has to admit the issue is real, and that you accept yourself despite the problem.
The phrase normally used goes like this:
'Even though I have this … (e.g. anger),
I deeply and completely accept myself.'
Change the phrase, where it says (e.g. anger), and insert the problem you want to address. Always use a problem that you have personally, and not someone else's.
If you feel anger at your partner because he has abused you, you wouldn't say;

'Even though he is abusive'

… but instead say …
'Even though I have this anger about his abuse'.
It always has to be an issue you have and not someone else.

Practise your phrase several times, until it runs off your tongue before you start the exercise;

'Even though I have this ... (pain, anger, guilt, shame, etc.) ... I deeply and completely accept myself'.

3. Tapping in Order
The Tapping Order usually covers nine meridian points.

1. Karate chop area (the side of the palm on the small finger side).
2. Eyebrows (the middle of each eyebrow).
3. Side of the eyes (in front of the temples).
4. Under the eyes (on the skull just below the eye socket).
5. Under the nose (the top of the top lip).
6. Chin (front of the chin).
7. The inner end of the collarbone (beside the neck).
8. Under the arm (on the side of the torso just below the bottom of the armpit).
9. The top of the head (crown).

Using the tips of the three middle fingers of each hand, tap on these points in turn (lifting the tips of the fingers about half an inch to an inch off the surface as you tap).

As you gently tap on the karate chop point with the three fingers on your other hand, say the phrase you learned above three times, out loud. Keep tapping while you repeat the phrase.

Then move on to tap each point **seven** times in the following order;

1. Eyebrow
2. Side of the eye
3. Under the eye

4. Under the nose
5. Chin
6. Inner end of the collarbone
7. Under the arm
8. At the top of the head

4. As you move down through the Tapping Points, recite a shorter version of your first phrase

If the first phrase is,

'Even although I have this anger, I deeply and completely accept myself'

your shorter version can be,

> *'This anger I feel because my partner is abusive.'*
> *'This anger I feel because my partner is abusive.'*
> *'This anger I feel because my partner is abusive.'*

- Recite this phrase while tapping each point seven times.
- Repeat the whole sequence two or three times.

5. Check how you feel after Tapping

After you repeat the exercise three times or more, ask yourself where your anxiety level is, from 0 to 10. Compare this level with the one before you did the Tapping. Ideally, you would like it to be 0, so if you have time, just keep repeating the exercise until you do. Repeat it throughout the day and keep aiming to reach 0 on the scale before the end of the day.

If you have other issues you want to work through, then substitute your 'problem' in the original phrase for your next issue.

Use Tapping when you become aware of overwhelming emotions or physical pain throughout the day.

Tapping is the last exercise in the book. Used in conjunction with the others, and if practised repeatedly, as described, you should soon feel self-confidence beginning to return. It may not be obvious at first, but there should be a shift in the way you see yourself and your situation, as the weeks go on. Trust and faith in yourself will return, as you start to make better decisions and begin looking at new possibilities for your future. Possibilities that you previously believed impossible.

No one else can do these exercises for you, the effort needed to cause the change in your mindset must come from *you*.

No one can do this for *you*. *You* must want this change, *you* must want a better, happier life and *you* must put the effort into these exercises to discover what they can deliver. If you do this, they will begin to change the way you see yourself and your vision of the future. Your mind will start to uncover ways to change the situations you previously thought were impossible to do anything about.

No one can tell you how good it will feel when the effects of these exercises begin to kick in. Have faith in the power they have to change your subconscious beliefs, and overcome the negative and debilitating effects DMA has had on your mind.

To know this and feel it for yourself, you have to make these exercises part of your life, no one else can do this for you, it's in your mind the changes have to happen, and it is with your conscious mind you have to practise them.

It will be worth it.

Here is a little bonus exercise, that is powerful enough to stand alone:

When you get the chance, pick up a pad of 'Post-it' notes. The little coloured square notepads with the sticky strip you can put just about anywhere, and at the same time get a thick black felt pen.
Now take the pad and pen, and wander about your house choosing random but prominent places to stick these little sheets of paper. Put them where you will come across them every day. It could be on the mirror in the bathroom, inside the cupboard that you keep your breakfast cereal in, inside a drawer, or even on the dashboard of your car, as long as it doesn't interfere with your driving.
Once you decide on a place to put each one, write on it, in capital letters …

I AM ENOUGH

Do as many as you can, so that you encounter several of them throughout the day and every time you see one, say out loud, 'I AM ENOUGH' three times.

That's it. The easiest exercise has been left till last.
You don't need to set alarms or timers for this, and you don't need to try to remember to do it either. You don't even need to make time to do it, because it takes no time to say, *'I am enough, I am enough, I am enough'*, whether it's as you look at yourself in the mirror or when you eat your cereal in the morning.

Do it, because, **'YOU ARE ENOUGH'**, you always have been, things in life just convinced you otherwise, until now.

CHAPTER 13

BRINGING IT ALL TOGETHER

Domestic mental abuse is a very difficult thing to recognise. Even when you are the one being abused.

Onlookers may notice when a woman's partner is treating her badly, but many of them don't realise what they are witnessing is actually domestic mental abuse. Nor do they realise that many of these men want to control every aspect of their partner's life, or the devastating effect this has on a woman's mind.

These men are so cunning, that very few people notice what they are doing to their partner's minds. Not many abusers show their hand at the beginning of a relationship, and very few will be silly enough to attempt to take over every aspect of your life right away. But slowly and surely they will spin their web, using lies, deception, trickery, charm and threat in equal measure to obtain what they desire. Eventually, many of them gain complete dominance over their partner's lives, and often, many women will have no idea how they ended up 'trapped' in that abusive situation.

These men manipulate your emotions while feeling little sympathy or empathy toward you. As they play with your feelings, you struggle to understand what is going on in your relationship. You may end up asking yourself, 'is it love, hate, fear, guilt, shame or jealousy that causes him to be like this?'

Unfortunately, these men are born with this type of personality, it's in their genes, and there is nothing you or anyone else can do to change it. They can't even change it themselves and many of them don't think there's anything wrong with the way they are acting. As they mentally manipulate you, they instil reasons and excuses that encourage you to stay with them in a life of downward spiralling misery. It can, in certain cases, be miserable for them too.

Some people will claim these individuals can change, but that argument has no material basis in fact, and history has taught us that. Usually, the idea of helping a mentally abusive man get over his 'illness', comes from those who have little personal experience of DMA themselves. They may have studied it in theory, but not experienced it in life. Like many subjects in reality, what is documented in textbooks can be a distant cousin to what happens in real life.

If anyone has managed to revive a DMA relationship to the point where the woman ends up with an equal say in it, they have kept it a closely guarded secret so far. There are millions of women around the world waiting for their partners to change and for the mental abuse to stop. Sadly though, that idea has been lodged in their mind by the very abuse they so desperately want to escape. Holding on to this thought gives the woman hope, and a reason to stay with her abuser, but all that stems from his conditioning and is all part of a long-term plan.

However, no matter how old you are, there is still a way to create long term happiness in the future, and it is outlined in this book.

Firstly, a woman has to recognise and accept she has fallen into an abusive relationship without realising it, but through no fault of her own.

Mental abusers are born with the ability to deceive the most intelligent and intuitive women and make them believe they are in a safe and cherished relationship. They will do this while undermining a woman's self-esteem, qualities and talents. This will all happen so surreptitiously, that she won't notice what she is caught up in.

One day, she will wake up with a feeling of dread and knots in her stomach, realising that there is something terribly wrong in her life. Even then, she is not likely to point the finger of suspicion at her partner. She might realise he has not been treating her as well as he used to. However, she probably won't realise that the way she sees the world has been altered by his manipulative influence.

How has he managed this, without her realising?

His genes contain the information to achieve this control of a partner, without physical violence. His chosen partner is up against knowledge handed down from the generations of mental abusers that came before him. His abilities to play with her thoughts and emotions come from information learned and perfected by past generations. That is how mental abuse is so effective, and why it is so successful.

It also has the perfect accomplice, that Trojan Horse in everyone's mind … the Inner Abuser.

The part of our mind that works against us, keeping us in a state of misery and suffering whenever it gets a chance to influence our thoughts and the decisions we make in our lives.

While we are not aware of it and the mental abuse in our relationship gets worse, our Inner Abuser gets stronger. Eventually, one day, we are so confused, our minds are so broken, that the Inner Abuser, aided by a daily helping of mental abuse from our partner takes almost complete control of our thoughts, actions and decision-making.

Even at this point in a relationship, we may still not recognise that what's going on is actually domestic mental abuse.

It's not only torment for the woman being abused, her family and friends that care for her are affected too. They are left feeling frustrated and powerless when they are unable to convince her she needs to escape her toxic partner.

THE TRUTH IS …

Once a woman realises she is being mentally abused by her partner it is better to leave him, if she ever wants to survive and thrive in life.

The problem is, mental abuse creates the illusion that the woman is still in control of her thoughts. Remember the woman who asked me, 'If I saw someone else being treated like this, I would tell them to run, and never look back, so why can't I?'.

It is possible to be so completely brainwashed, that you are unable to deal with the idea that your partner is, for all intents and purposes, 'in control of your mind, your beliefs, and your decisions'.

Trying to convince someone in this state of mind is like asking them to cross a minefield to freedom when they think they are free already. They don't see the point of the exercise.

They don't think there is a need to fight mental abuse when they don't believe they're being mentally abused.

Reading this book may help convince some women they are not free and that they need some help to get across that 'minefield' after all.

ONCE AWAKE TO THE DECEPTION …

…there is a way back, but like any journey, it starts with the first step. When a woman realises she is in an abusive relationship, there may be a period of shock and bewilderment, before the gravity of the situation sinks in.

Once it does, there can be a desperate desire to escape right away. This is part of the reason so many women leave their abusive partners only to return to them time and time again. They are not prepared mentally, for what's to come, and it's not usually a successful time to try to escape.

TO SUCCEED IT'S BEST TO MAKE A PLAN ...

... I know it sounds daunting but you might want to read this book over again, especially if you didn't mark all the things that are more important to you personally. Become aware of your Inner Abuser. Think about the influence it had on decisions you made in the past. Recognise the ones that have caused you the biggest problems. Learn from that, and try to be more vigilant of your thoughts from now on. Think about the consequences making wrong decisions in the future could have. Try to slow down and be careful that the Inner Abuser does not influence your decisions from now on. Realise you need to be extra careful, until you strengthen your mind with the help of this book. Accept that the Inner Abuser, fuelled by DMA is still the strongest part of your mind at the moment.

Begin working with the exercises in this book every day. Turn them into a habit and allow them time to strengthen your mind. Do this consistently and you will break the hold the Inner Abuser and DMA have on your thoughts and decision making.

The power to change your circumstances and take back control of your life lies with you, not your abusive partner. DMA has clouded your ability to make good decisions for yourself ... **UNTIL NOW ...**

... as you work with these exercises, belief in yourself will return, the ability to recognise your partner as an abusive individual will surface and the realisation you need to leave him will present itself naturally. But not in the heat of the moment, only when you are calm and in control of your thoughts and your plan is in place. This book was never about learning to live with him, I don't recommend staying with a mentally abusive individual, because in time, they only ever get worse, never better. You cannot change him and your goal can only be achieved when you work to change yourself.

WHEN THE TIME IS RIGHT

Once you have clarity and control of your thoughts, his words and actions will no longer affect you the way they once did and you will feel strong enough to put your plan to leave into action. Leave when he is not around and you won't be hampered getting out of the house for the last time. If you discuss leaving with him, it is likely that you will not find it easy to walk away. These abusers are very good at convincing you they will change, and because you have been influenced by his DMA, there's every chance you might capitulate, even at that late stage of a plan.

Like Jason avoiding the Gorgon's stare, you must leave when he is not around and avoid being turned to 'stone' too.

Follow the recommendations for leaving him safely in the two parts of Chapter 9.

Take all the advice in this book seriously and do not underestimate what he might do once you have left. There is a big chance he will go all out to find you, confront you and entice or force you back with him. He will also resort to pleading and crying his eyes out if it obtains the desired effect.

Ideally, you should only leave when you are 'over him' in your mind, after that his words will have little effect on you. If you find you can't wait any longer, and living with him has become too dangerous, try to repeat the exercises as often as you can, before, during and after the time you walk out the front door for the last time.

Follow the advice and leave quickly with a minimum of fuss.

Once in your new accommodation, you can congratulate yourself, there may be challenges ahead, but if you continue the exercises regularly, you will find the strength to deal with any difficulties that present themselves.

NO (WO)MAN'S LAND

Once you have left him, your life may feel unusual for a while. To begin with, you will not be living with a constant barrage of abuse every day and this lack of drama will feel strangely uncomfortable. This is perfectly normal, even when that situation was not good for you. The human brain 'craves' what it has been used to, that's why most of us don't like change. It's also why we become attached to things and it is even possible to get attached to abuse.

This slightly bewildering, sometimes unnerving feeling will pass over a period of time, but it's important to know it can happen. Any thoughts that appear of you returning to him should be dismissed by using one of the exercises to divert your attention onto something more positive for the future. A day will come when you will begin to enjoy your newfound freedom, without negative thoughts and full of possibilities for the future. What people and places will you discover in your new life?

At some point, even if you follow all this advice, you may have to deal with your ex if he finds out where you live and turns up at your door. How much you feel you have to prepare for this will determine how secure you feel in your new home.

Regardless of what does or doesn't happen, it is best **never** to communicate with him directly again, even if you feel you are able to deal with him in the future.

Be careful not to fall into this trap. Remember, your Inner Abuser will always be in the background, languishing in your subconscious, trying to create drama and undermine the progress you make with this book. Having no direct communication with him is one of the most important decisions you can make.

AVOID HIM OR REPORT HIM

If you don't come to terms with this choice, your ex may torment you for years, finding any 'legitimate' reason he can to contact you through any means he can. More importantly, if you have a nagging doubt about this, he will remain in your subconscious, appearing in random thoughts, out of the blue, to disrupt your new life and if you want to beat the effects of DMA, you don't want that to happen.

FINALLY …

To ensure you enjoy life to the full after a DMA relationship I urge you to continue to use these exercises regularly.

You might be happy to reduce the number of times a week you spend with them, but you should continue to do so regularly, to maintain the most positive mindset you can. But, if you notice your Inner Abuser creating negative waves, or influencing you to make bad decisions you should immediately return to practising them every day.

One of the lingering shadows of a long-term DMA relationship is the inability to have a kind, caring, sharing and loving relationship after surviving such an experience. However, continuing to work with the exercises after escaping his persistent advances will help to minimise any memories you have about your ex, being transferred onto any future partner. It is perfectly normal to be cautious, but it is also possible to build a new relationship with the right person and ignore fears from the past. A new relationship can be based on trust, love and equality.

One other thing to look out for … be careful **you** don't end up showing signs of mental abuse towards a new partner. Having lived with a mental abuser for a long period, you may have unconsciously picked up his traits, and may end up portraying them yourself, in a new relationship.

Monitor the way you communicate with a new partner and be careful you don't subconsciously show any signs of control or mental abuse towards them.

It may sound strange, but when it was a 'normal' part of your previous relationship, your subconscious may still think it's acceptable in a new one.

This could be a subliminal act of self-defence, but if you continue to work with this book, building and improving the confidence you have in yourself, it will help to reassure you there is no need to feel dominant, either consciously or subconsciously.

₪

No matter how much help you seek from others or no matter how much help you get from others, to beat DMA you must ultimately do it yourself. This is an abuse of **your** mind, in **your** mind and the only one that is in a position to reverse **your** mind is **you**. Of course, it is always worth calling on good, trustworthy people around you to give you support when times are tough. Use that support and the information in this book, knowing there will come a day when you regain the strength of mind and the determination to create a better life for yourself. A much better life than you could have if you remain in a relationship with a narcissist.

YOU HAVE THE POWER TO DEAL WITH DMA INSIDE YOU, YOU JUST NEED TO GO IN THERE AND DISCOVER IT FOR YOURSELF

A word of caution:
The Inner Abuser will never disappear completely, it is part of you. We all have an Inner Abuser, but as long as we learn to recognise its influence and deal with that early enough, we can ensure a much better life for ourselves in the future.

Even the best of us, the late great Louise Hay, founder of the Hay House organisation, spoke of times when she would feel the need to return to do mirror work with her reflection until she felt better, and she was still doing it all the way through her long life. Even into her eighties.

We all have an Inner Abuser, not just those of us who have been affected by mental abuse, every one of us should take some time to check inwards, to make sure we are not being manipulated by that insatiable part of our mind that's always trying to convince us to make bad decisions.

Like anything in life, it's only when you know something exists that you can do anything about it. No matter how successful you are at leaving a DMA relationship behind, I urge you to make these exercises a part of your life from now on. Every day you enjoy from now on, will make you glad you did.

You have the power to create your own future and make it a good one.

CHAPTER 14

... AND FINALLY

There is a good reason why the title on the following page is the last subject in this book, you should return to the start of the exercises and continue to re-read all the points you underlined or highlighted when you read through the book for the first time.

I will ask you not to read this last chapter until you have used the exercises regularly for several weeks and have felt a shift in the way you see your life. By the time you decide you are ready to turn the next page of this book, you should be well away from your abusive partner and already rebuilding a happier and less stressful life.

That is what this book was created to do. If you are not quite there yet, go back and continue working with the exercises for another few weeks before reading beyond this page.

Make a note in the margin to remind yourself that only when you are ready, and after you have left your abusive partner and when your mind feels clear and strong, then and only then should you turn the page and read this final chapter ...

CHAPTER 15

FORGIVENESS

Over the years, the idea of forgiveness has been misinterpreted. When we discuss forgiving someone, many of us believe we are relinquishing them of any blame attached to their wrongdoings, but we're not. We are releasing the bitterness and grudge we hold inside us, towards that individual. We are deciding that we will not continue to harbour a grievance towards them any further. We are not absolving them of their actions, we are simply deciding to let go of the feelings those actions have created in us.

But to forgive anyone else, we have to forgive ourselves first.

- Forgive ourselves for the perception we previously had of our lives.
- Forgive ourselves for anything we felt guilty about.
- Forgive ourselves for allowing the situation we felt trapped in to continue for so long.

Forgiveness is something more though, it means we are no longer fighting the source of our bitterness, we are letting it go. In essence, we are surrendering to it, which means we are no longer battling with it … and that means it no longer has any power over us and we can walk away from it.

The past is gone, no matter how long we analyse it, regret it or feel guilty about it, it is gone. We cannot go back and change it, and therefore it no longer serves us to continue pondering over it. Any time you find yourself thinking 'what if' or 'if only', remind yourself, that this thought process does not serve you. By regularly repeating the exercises we learn to forget the details of past events. The only thing we should retain is the lessons we learned from them. All else is a misuse of our mind, and when we misuse our mind, we can slip back into the realms of our Inner Abuser.

Once we achieve that act of self-forgiveness, that act of surrender, we can do the one thing that will set us free from the prison DMA creates in our minds … and learn how to forgive the man that caused us so much sorrow.

Forgiving does not mean allowing him back into your mind or your life, indeed it is the exact opposite, you are ready to release him from your mind. He no longer has any power over your thoughts and emotions and the way they make you feel. Hearing his name does not cause you distress, regret, guilt or fear, and you remain neutral if someone else brings it up.

As time goes by, people will accept that you no longer wish to discuss him, for good or bad. They will realise you will not tolerate his company, more because you know the kind of individual he is, and not so much because of your past experiences with him. In the fullness of time, once you have explained the situation, those around you will come to understand that if he were to approach you in the future, you have to protect yourself, and the best way to do that is by contacting the authorities.

Once you forgive him in your mind, try to forget about him. When you can honestly say you rarely think about him, and if you do, it has no impact on your mood, you will know that any hold he did have over your mind and your life has gone. For more information, please visit and share the website with others you think may benefit from this book.

domesticmentalabuse.com

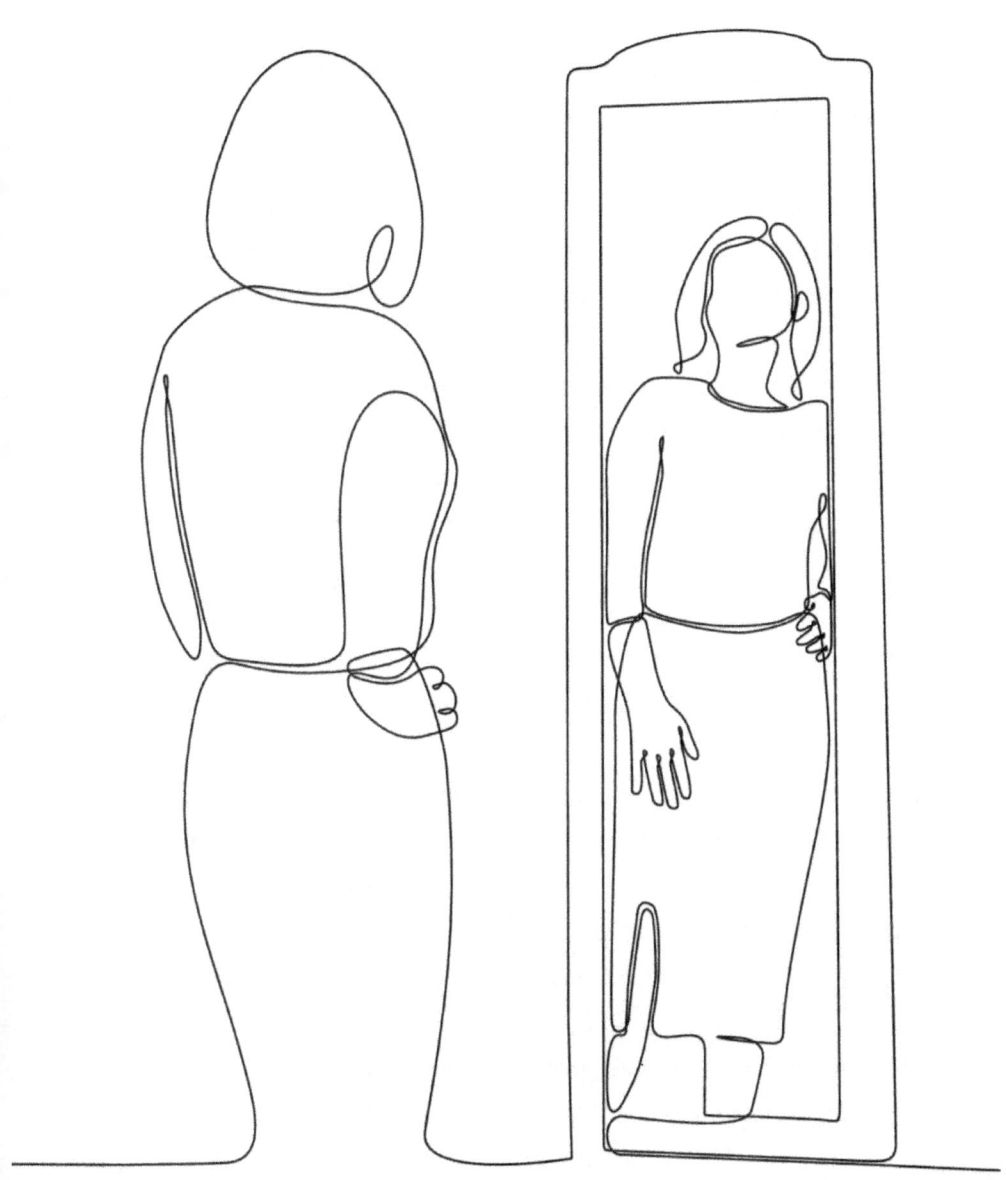

DISCLAIMER AND TERMS OF USE AGREEMENT

The author has used their best efforts in creating these materials. No representation or warranties are made concerning the accuracy, applicability, or sufficiency of the contents of those materials.

The information contained herein is strictly for educational purposes. Therefore, if you would like to apply the ideas contained in these materials, you're taking full responsibility for your actions.

Every effort has been made to accurately represent these materials, the contents, and their potential. However, there's no guarantee that you will improve in any way using the techniques and ideas in these materials, and examples in these materials aren't to be interpreted as a promise of anything or a guarantee of anything.

Self-help and improvement potential is entirely hooked in to the person using these materials, ideas and techniques.

Your level of improvement in achieving the results claimed in these materials depends on the time you devote to the programme, ideas and techniques mentioned. Individuals' knowledge and skills differ therefore we cannot guarantee anyone's success. Nor be held liable for any of your actions.

There are not any guarantees given or implied concerning any results you may or may not achieve from our ideas and techniques in this material.

The author disclaims any warranties (express or implied), merchantability or fitness for any particular purpose.

The author shall in no event be held susceptible to any party for any direct, indirect, punitive, special, incidental or other consequential damages arising directly or indirectly from any use of this material, which is provided 'as is', and without warranties.

As always, a competent professional's advice should be sought. The author don't warrant the performance, effectiveness or applicability of any sites listed or linked to in these materials. All links are for information purposes only and aren't warranted for content, accuracy or the other implied or explicit purpose.